Survivor Blessings:
My Breast Cancer Story

Shelley Chase

Published by FernAcres Publishing

Survivor Blessings:

My Breast Cancer Story

Shelley Chase

About This Book

In 2008, I received a diagnosis of breast cancer. It changed my life.

At the time, I was too overwhelmed to journal, or blog, or even post many status updates on my brand new Facebook account. But now, five years have passed, and after reflecting on the lessons and the blessings I unexpectedly received, I feel it is time to share this journey. It is my hope that someone else who has just been diagnosed, or is going through treatment, can be encouraged by reading about my breast cancer adventure.

Since my email server has been so kind as to save all the email messages I sent out five years ago, I am able to tell the story as it unfolds in my life. This is the story of friends and relatives stepping up to bless our family, and the story of how our family learned to set aside our pride and gratefully receive those blessings. It is a story of how God held me in His right hand.

A word of caution here: thanks to the internet, there is no end of stories about other people's cancers, and how they are treated, and what can go wrong. My story is no different...in fact, it may even be a rare case of "if it can go wrong, it will." If you are about to go through this yourself, or if you are preparing to help out a loved one, then please overlook all the difficulties and focus on the encouragement, love, and blessings that can be received. This is a story of hope! It has been more than 5 years since I was diagnosed, and I remain (as far as I know) cancer-free. And as my surgeon once told me, I can now sit with my friends over a cup of coffee and enjoy the fact that the journey is long behind me.

Cast of characters:

Since the emails are sent to and from a large assortment of people, I should probably introduce them to you, as they were in 2008:

Me: Stay-at-home mom who has homeschooled my kids for 10 years.

Eric: my husband, who is awesome and my hero.

Sharon and Kristin: daughters 18 and 21, who at the time were both in college. Sharon was engaged to Will, and their wedding was scheduled for June of 2008, just three months after my diagnosis.

Andy and Luke: sons 15 and 9. Andy attended a high school across town. Luke was my only homeschool student.

House Church: Two weeks before my diagnosis, we started holding a house church in our home every Wednesday night, for prayer and Bible study. These were a new group of folks from our church, who were just meeting and getting to know each other.

Cindy: My sister, who had just moved up to Oregon from California with her family.

Karen and Loyal: My brother and his wife, who lived in California

Gini, Cami, Tanya, Vicki, Marlene: Some of the amazing friends who supported me. They were part of a small group Bible study that our families had been doing for many years.

Mike: We started a major remodeling of our house in July of 2007, which was almost complete. Mike was the contractor, but during the remodel, also become a friend.

Karla: She was the landscape architect who helped us choose plants for our newly landscaped garden. Her mom had just passed away from breast cancer.

Sylvia and Bill: My future son-in-law's parents

Diagnosis

During the summer of 2007 I was due for my mammogram. I was 44 years old and none of my relatives had ever had breast cancer. I'd had three previous mammograms, all clean. I had never felt a lump, although I had for months felt a little itchy in one spot. With no risk factors for breast cancer, I really didn't feel the urgency to go get the "big squeeze". We were up to our knees in remodeling dust and debris, and I was busy. So I put it off. For six months. No big deal.

After I finally went to the appointment, they left me in that little room with the curtain for a long time. They must be busy, I reasoned.

Finally, the nurse came back and said they needed to redo one of the pictures. Still not worried.

After another long wait in the little cotton gown, the nurse came to tell me that the doctor wanted to do an ultrasound on one area on the left side. Since they just happened to not be busy (could have fooled me, I thought) they could do it immediately. During the ultrasound, the doctor reassured me, telling me it looked like the blob they saw was just a cyst. But there were two tiny areas, very small, just behind the cyst. You couldn't even see them on the mammogram. It was probably nothing. But he wanted to do a biopsy.

From: Shelley
Sent: Wednesday, March 05, 2008 10:15 AM
To: Tanya, Gini, Cami
Subject: Prayers please

OK, ladies:

Prayer here please:

I have to go in for a biopsy on Monday for two lumps they discovered during my mammogram this week...that's right, the mammogram I had put off for 6 months! Anyway, I'm not too worried at this point, the doc said one of them is probably just a cyst, but appreciate lots of prayer for peace and good test results. I am so thankful it's me and not one of the kids this time!

Shelley

From: Cami
Sent:Wednesday, March 05, 2008 8:11 PM
To:Shelley
Subject: Re: Prayers please

Praying here Shelley! I remember those same feelings when I had a surgical biopsy.

Heavenly Father, Please bring comfort and peace to Shelley as she waits through this process. May you guide the drs. and bring the exact diagnosis on what is going on in her body. We trust in you for all that you want to accomplish in her precious life. In Jesus name, Amen.

Biopsy day came. According to my exhaustive internet searches, biopsies were awful, painful, and scary. I wanted to go by myself. But the nurse said I wouldn't be able to drive home afterwards, so I reluctantly agreed to let my husband drive me. I just didn't want to bother him during a weekday!

With a little help from some valium (highly recommend this!), the biopsy was much easier than I expected. They numbed me up, and I got to watch them take the sample on the ultrasound monitor. This was pretty cool. I was a science teacher before kids, and medical stuff fascinates me.

The doctor said he thought he removed all of both tumors just from the biopsies, they were so small. I told him to take as much as he wanted to, no need to leave anything behind. He inserted a small metal marker where the lumps used to be, just to help find the spot again if needed. But, he assured me, the spots just looked like cysts. They were probably nothing to worry about.

From: Shelley Chase
Sent: Monday, March 10, 2008 2:42 PM
To: Cami; Gini; Vicki; Marlene; Tanya; Cindy
Subject: all done
Hi ladies:
Biopsy was a piece of cake, pretty painless actually, and interesting! I got to watch as they did things on the ultrasound. Took stuff from two lumps, won't know anything until late Wednesday. Doing fine and resting comfortably numb now, although they gave me a prescription for Vicadin, so I can pretty much guess what's coming.

Thanks for the prayers and keep them coming!

Shelley

From: Marlene
Sent: Tuesday, March 11, 2008 10:33 AM
To: Shelley
Subject: Re: all done

On my way home last night I realized that I may have sounded a bit hasty – making it sound like you "had" breast cancer. What I was meaning was that in finding the lump and having the biopsy procedure, I'm interested in how things go with the new technology. Lots of things have changed over the years since 1986 and 1998. I have my mammogram tomorrow – and have noticed over the last 4 or 5 years they are less painful – since they heightened the sensitivity of the machines.

I'm going to just assume everything is benign. How ya feeling today?

Marlene

From: Shelley Chase
Sent: Monday, March 10, 2008 2:42 PM
To: Marlene
Subject: Re: all done

No worries here, God led me to Psalm 91 yesterday, and I'm hiding behind His feathers from the deadly pestilence :)

You're right, the technology is much improved. The ultrasound lady was saying that they probably wouldn't have seen anything at all or been able to locate the lumps on any lesser of a machine than they had. Apparently some places have older machines that wouldn't be able to see such small lumps (<1 cm). Also the mammograms are all digital now (at least at this place) which is better, I'm assuming.

I am just a little bit sore today, haven't needed any pain meds other than the Tylenol yesterday. Know where I could go to sell a bunch of Vicadin on the streets? (Just kidding, all email interceptors!! I would never break the law!!)

Shelley

Psalm 91

Whoever dwells in the shelter of the Most High
   will rest in the shadow of the Almighty.
I will say of the Lord, "He is my refuge and my fortress,
   my God, in whom I trust."

Surely he will save you
   from the fowler's snare
   and from the deadly pestilence.
He will cover you with his feathers,
   and under his wings you will find refuge;
   his faithfulness will be your shield and rampart.
You will not fear the terror of night,
   nor the arrow that flies by day,
nor the pestilence that stalks in the darkness,
   nor the plague that destroys at midday.
A thousand may fall at your side,
   ten thousand at your right hand,
   but it will not come near you.
You will only observe with your eyes
   and see the punishment of the wicked.

If you say, "The Lord is my refuge,"
   and you make the Most High your dwelling,
no harm will overtake you,

no disaster will come near your tent.
For he will command his angels concerning you
to guard you in all your ways;
they will lift you up in their hands,
so that you will not strike your foot against a stone.
You will tread on the lion and the cobra;
you will trample the great lion and the serpent.

"Because he loves me," says the Lord, "I will rescue him;
I will protect him, for he acknowledges my name.
He will call on me, and I will answer him;
I will be with him in trouble,
I will deliver him and honor him.
With long life I will satisfy him
and show him my salvation." NIV

From: Marlene
Sent: Monday, March 10, 2008 2:51 PM
To: Shelley Chase
Subject: RE: all done
Give yourself some TLC. Ouch! I know someday I'll have to have
that done, so I'm going to watch you and see how it goes. Both of
my sisters had breast cancer, but it's been a few years, and
technology has improved. Take care of yourself !!!
Marlene

From: Cindy
Sent: Monday, March 10, 2008 7:59 PM
To: Cindy
Subject: Re: all done
Hi Shell,
Thanks for the update. I was praying for you all day.

Love,
Cindy

Two days later, we had a late afternoon appointment to get the results of the biopsy. It seemed to take forever to get there! Bad traffic, trains, road work...by the time we made it there, ten minutes late, I was pretty stressed out. I really hate being late.

Of course, then we had to wait for the doctor. And wait. Finally he came in and told us that they had trouble finding the test results. He had glanced over them quickly, almost sure the biopsies had come up clean.

He was
wrong.

From: Shelley
Sent: Wednesday, March 12, 2008 6:22 PM
To: Cindy
Subject: biopsy results
Hi Cindy:

In a hurry because of house church tonight, but here is the info in order of importance:

curable
early stage
no chemo probably, just radiation

Thanks so much for your prayers!! The doc couldn't believe how calm I was. I had an inkling this was coming, not sure why. I'll update you with more info as we get it.

Shelley

From: Cindy
Sent:Wednesday, March 12, 2008 10:43 PM
To: Shelley
Subject: Re:biopsy results
Hi Shell,

 Thanks for not making me wait till tomorrow. I prayed non-stop as I
was at the Y from 4 to 5. After what you said about the biopsy
today, I guess I knew then. I will definitely tell Mom tomorrow. I'll go
over there in the morning. I will just let her know how Steve felt and
wanted to be treated when he went through chemo and radiation. I
know that you will get through this just fine. I am here to help
anyway you need while you go through treatments. If you want me
to pick up and take the boys places, or do homeschool with Luke on
days you don't feel up to it, whatever, I am here. We have an
amazing God!!!

He brought us up here, because he already knew that you would
need family nearby.

 Love you   .
Cindy

After the appointment, my husband and I hurried home to get the
house ready for house church. This was only our second meeting
and we hadn't yet got the routine down for making coffee, setting
out the snacks, and arranging the chairs.

We discussed whether or not we should tell everyone the news. We
barely knew these people! Do I really want a bunch of strangers
worrying about me? Should we tell them?

I decided to just play it by ear. Wait and see how the night went. See how many other people had big prayer requests. Mine was not that urgent.

But I did share. When the leader asked if there were any prayer needs, I spoke up and explained how hours ago I had been diagnosed with breast cancer. Immediately, people jumped up and surrounded me, laid hands on me, prayed for my healing. I felt so incredibly blessed. We wouldn't have to go through this alone!

I was still afraid, though. My family needed me! Why would God put my life in danger when my kids still needed me so much? The next day I took my Bible and demanded some answers. As I sometimes do, I let my Bible fall open. This is the first thing I read:

Because you are my help,
I sing in the shadow of your wings.

My soul clings to you;
your right hand upholds me.

They who seek my life will be destroyed;
they will go down to the depths of the earth.[2]

No way! I tried again.

Save us and help us with your right hand,
that those you love may be delivered.[3]

By now, tears were flowing. I turned over a couple of pages and pointed randomly again.

Though I walk in the midst of trouble,
you preserve my life;
you stretch out your hand against the anger of my foes,
with your right hand you save me.[4]

Well, then. The words of the psalmist came right from God to me. God's right hand would save me, deliver me, uphold me. It was going to be
OK.

From: Shelley
Sent:Thursday, March 13, 2008 3:58 PM
To: Marlene
Subject: RE:biopsy results
Hi Marlene:

All I could find today reading the Bible were verses about God holding me in his right hand.

I was able to get an appointment with a surgeon tomorrow, hurray for speediness, so I'll know then when the surgery will be. Radiation will start two weeks after.

Specific prayer requests: that the surgeon will have time to do the surgery next week. We are only 14 weeks from the wedding and about 10 of that will be surgery and radiation. Also, if that happens, that I can postpone our Colorado plane tickets without too much of a $ penalty. We were supposed to be gone next M-Th. Protection from the evil one: someone worked very hard not to get us to that appointment yesterday, but because we were able to get results before they closed, House church people were able to pray last night.

Thanks so much!! I appreciate the info since I don't personally know anyone who has gone through this.

Shelley

From: Marlene
Sent:Friday, March 14, 2008 10:14 AM
To: Shelley
Subject: Re:biopsy results

I would suggest you ask your professionals about the tiredness and if there are any specific "stress" vitamins you could take during that time. It's best to take things up front so that you can save yourself getting tired first, then trying to climb the hill of tiredness after it has started. Then again, you may not be bothered with that, but I have heard other radiation patients mention it. Then if you think about it, the stress of the daily treatments, going to and from your appointments, and everything you need to do and not do surrounding that issue, can definitely make one tired.

Also, I know they gave my sister some kind of cream for the redness and extreme tenderness, but she was still pretty sore. Are these little lumps in the same breast or one in each?...if you said it, I don't recall.

My prayers are with you, and if you ever need any help, please let me know. Take good care of yourself – during this phase YOU "must" come first.

God Bless!!!!

Marlene

From: Shelley
Sent:Friday, March 14, 2008 8:15 AM
To: Mike
Subject: Under attack again
Hi Mike:

This time the girls are both safe, no grandma issues, the attack is on me (and I suppose everyone else in the family is affected too, come to think of it). Diagnosed this week with breast cancer. It's a really early stage, so supposedly very curable, but I need surgery and radiation. Hoping to get all this done soon because only 14 weeks to wedding!! At least I have a beautiful (and completed!) house to recuperate in.

Prayers much appreciated! Meeting with a surgeon today to set date.

Thanks!

Shelley

From: Shelley
Sent:Friday, March 14, 2008 2:43 PM
To: Mike
Subject: Re: Under attack again
OK, God is good. Because I was able to get in to see the surgeon today, I was able to move my MRI up to Tuesday and get surgery next Thursday. Otherwise it would have been another two weeks. Maybe in about two weeks, dinner would be much appreciated! Thanks so much for the prayers, I am not anxious about the outcome of this at all.

From: Shelley
Sent:Friday, March 14, 2008 3:24 PM
To: Sylvia and Bill
Subject: Sorry!
Hi Sylvia and Bill:

I guess Will has updated you on the news...so sorry to miss out on the shower fun! I'm not sure what we'll do with those airplane tickets, that will be the next thing to figure out.

No worries here, God has me in His hand. I am so glad I could get in to see the surgeon so quickly and that we can get this process started and completed before the wedding. They think about 10-12 weeks from surgery to end of radiation (probably no chemo needed). Since we have about 14 weeks until the wedding, it's cutting it a little close, but it should be fine. Surgery will be this next Thursday afternoon.

Maybe you and Sharon and Will can discuss making the "bird-seed" bags for people to throw, and figure out the wedding favors? That would be a great help. Not too much else to plan on this end, I think the caterer and the photographer have everything figured out.

Thanks for your prayers, greatly appreciated!!

love,

Shelley

My appointment with the surgeon was uneventful. She was very encouraging, telling me that the kind of breast cancer I had was very curable, more than 98%. She explained about lumpectomies, where she would just take out the offending tissue and a small margin around it. I wouldn't even need to stay overnight. I'd be home and resting by dinner time!

After that, I would probably need daily doses of radiation for a couple of months, just to make sure the spot was gone.

Daily? I had to go in for DAILY treatments? For months? I had a son to teach! I had a wedding to plan! But I guess it could be worse. 98% cure rate was pretty good.

And God was holding me in his right
hand.

Hi all:

God is so amazing, and I keep coming across scriptures (and people
keep giving me these same scriptures without knowing this!)
that tell me that He is holding me in His hand...a song even came on
the radio that said just that as I hopped out of the car for the
doctor's appointment Friday. Anyway, here is the update:

I was able to get in to see the surgeon for a consult Friday morning
(amazing that it was so quick). She was terrific and explained
everything thoroughly. With her help, we were able to move the
MRI up to this Tuesday (amazing they had an opening), and she will
be able to do the surgery on Thursday (amazing again that she had
an opening, since Good Friday pushes her surgery day up a
day). We'll know more after the MRI, but the doc says it looks
uncomplicated. Because of the kind and my age (unusually young
for this...HA...something I'm young for!) she will sample lymph
nodes just in case.

More amazing-ness: both of my girls will be coming home from
college for spring break at the end of the week, so I will have some
help. Plus, since the week after the surgery is spring break, I won't
have all the usual mom-driving duties. Even more amazing-ness:
the doc said you couldn't see any lumps on the mammogram. Only
a very close cyst caught their attention, which led to the ultrasound, which led to finding the other (very small) lump. Also, since I

had delayed getting this mammogram for 6 months (ahem, not an excuse for you, ladies) they were able to find it sooner. Six months ago it would have been too small to detect, so it would have been another six months from now that they found it. Assuming I didn't put off that mammogram either. Amazing.

Specific prayer requests: that the MRI on Tuesday doesn't show any cancer anywhere else, and things go smoothly on Thursday.

I have to tell you too, in light of the sermon today, how hard the evil one tried to prevent Eric and I from getting to the doctor on Wednesday in time to get the biopsy results. Despite train crossing delays, traffic jams, road work, a last minute call from Eric's boss, and missing test results, we made it to the appointment in time to get the results and get back home in time for house church. So we could pray right away!! Thanks so much for your prayers!! I really am doing just fine right now because of them!!

So, maybe much more detail than you-all need, but there you go. God is amazing!!

Shelley

From: Pam
Sent:Sunday, March 16, 2008 11:17 AM
To: Shelley
Subject: Re: Chase Update
Shelley,

I am so glad you sent this update. John said he talked with you & Eric this morning but I kept pumping him for more information than he had. :) You have been on my mind so much and I have been praying for you and Eric and your kids. On our drive home Wednesday night I couldn't imagine the heaviness of your hearts and not having time to even process it yet. I was also very thankful we were all able to pray for you. It sounds like scripture and prayer is how God is carrying you through. We are praising God with you for how quickly your MRI and surgery has been scheduled. He is so good!

I talked with Vickie at church this morning and she said they already told you they are offering their home as a back up as needed. Aren't they just the most loving people? I'm sure John & Anne would be willing as well if it's needed. Also, the Hallams would probably be an option as well. I'm very glad your daughters will be home for your recovery. I'm sure they are too.

As you will hear a lot, PLEASE let us know when we can help in any way. John & I will keep you in our prayers!

Pam

From: Shelley
Sent:Monday, March 17, 2008 9:11 AM
To: Pam
Subject: Re: Chase Update
Thanks, Pam. We'll let you know if we need to change houses, but my gut feeling on this is it will probably be just fine to keep having it here. All I really have to do is make coffee and tell the kids to put their stuff away! (they always do it so gladly, of course, wink, wink).

From: Shelley
Sent:Friday, March 14, 2008 2:50 PM
To: Cami, Gini, Tanya, Marlene, Cindy
Subject: Speediness Praise!
OK, God is good. Because I was able to get in to see the surgeon today, I was able to move my MRI up to Tuesday and get surgery next Thursday. Otherwise it would have been another two weeks. I like the surgeon; she took time to explain everything thoroughly. We'll know more after the MRI and the surgery about what we're

dealing with, but she told me, "Someday, you'll be sitting around having coffee with your friends and remembering the long ago cancer you went through. No need to worry that this will not be cured completely."

Shelley

From: Marlene
Sent:Friday, March 14, 2008 2:58 PM
To: Shelley
Subject: Re:Speediness Praise!
You WILL be a survivor!!!!! You will be able to wear the pink cap and pink shirt very proudly and be a testimony to other women about the benefits of regular mammograms and gyn visits. When you are watching your grandchildren become teenagers, then later as parents themselves, you will be so glad you had your mammogram!!!!!

Can you tell in the late 90's I was on the American Cancer Societies "Breast Cancer Awareness, Outreach and Education" Advisory Board? I did it in honor of the sister I lost to this disease. I don't want to lose any more women out of my life to this. I'm soooooo proud of you!!!!!

Marlene

From: Gini
Sent: Friday, March 14, 2008 6:22 PM
To: Shelley
Subject: Re: Speediness Praise!
Shelley,

God is good...Would you like help with MRI driving, Luke watching, meals??? What does the surgery entail? Are you in the hospital for long? I, like Cami, am looking forward to the coffee with friends.

praying and praying...we'll work out the Seder another time... let's see how you're feeling.

gini

From: Shelley
Sent: Saturday, Mar 15, 2008 at 9:47 AM
To: Gini
Subject: Re: Speediness Praise!
Luke watching would be a real blessing on Tuesday...not sure what your schedule is like, but the MRI starts at 11:20, so I would need to drop him off about 10:40. It is supposed to last 90 minutes, so it might be 1:30 or later for pick up. Would this work for you?

Surgery is supposed to just be a day-thing, depending on what they end up doing (which they find out in the middle of the surgery! Nothing like surprises.) I should be home late Thursday night, though.

From: Gini
Sent: Saturday, March 15, 2008 11:45 AM
To: Shelley
Subject: Re: Speediness Praise!
Luke is mine! Bring him sooner if you like as you might want to be there with enough time to catch your breath...or maybe not! I'd love to have him on Thursday as well...I'll make sure the family has dinner as well. I will work with your schedule. Of course, we'll want to be at the hospital if that works out. Just whatever is best for you, my friend. Praying... Psalm 61 and 62... You have some wonderful promises to hang on to. I'd type them in but we have a dress rehearsal in an hour or so.

love and praying, praying...

Gini

From: Shelley
Sent: Sunday, March 16, 2008 1:27 PM
To: Gini
Subject: Re: Speediness Praise!
Thanks, Gini!! Kristin and her friend will be home on Thursday, so I am thinking she will want to take the boys to Godfathers...that is their favorite thing to do. Eric will probably get something at the hospital. Can we raincheck that dinner to the following week? Sharon goes back to school on Tuesday, so that would be a great day, or any other day that week. Thanks so much.

How did the musical go today? We really wanted to come, but the day got away from us. Sharon has a concert at 4, so we are taking Grandma, then out to a birthday dinner after for her. I am sure the musical went great as it always does, no matter what happens. Hearts are touched!!

I have been madly doing as much as I can around here since I am thinking this will be my last good weekend for awhile :) (Hey, know any good movies? I might be needing some about this time next week...)

Shelley

From: Shelley
Sent: Tuesday, March 18, 2008 3:48 PM
To: Cami
Subject: Re: Speediness Praise!
Surgery tomorrow at noon, Good Sam. It was moved up because the surgeon was busy, not because of any pressing need. The MRI went well, nothing "jumped out" to the doc who gave it a quick once over before we left. He will examine it more this afternoon so that the surgeon has all the info she needs.

A meal Friday or Saturday would be fabulous! Everyone will be home, so six. Thank you, thank you!!

[2] Psalm 63:7-9

[3] Psalm 108:6

[4] Psalm 138:7

Surgery

From: Eric
Sent: Wednesday, March 17, 2008 8:02 PM
To: House Church
Subject: Chase Update
From Eric:

I wanted to send out a brief update of Shelley's status.

Shelley underwent lumpectomy surgery today and is now home resting. The surgeon said there were no signs of growth outside of the two lumps that they found last week. They also checked her lymph nodes and preliminarily the results are also good. We know you prayed for this outcome regarding Shelley's diagnosis and this is an answer to those prayers. Going into today (and through the MRI yesterday) Shelley has felt a real sense of calm, which is also an answer to your prayers. Thank you for lifting her up so faithfully.

She is still a little groggy and sore, so pain medication will be helpful for the coming days. There is also a radiation regimen coming up in a few weeks so your continued prayers for comfort and healing are greatly appreciated.

Andy, Luke and I are also being ministered to by many of you and I also thank you for that. My two daughters will be home in a few days and they will be a great blessing at this time as well.

May God bless you all
--
Eric Chase

From: Shelley
Sent: Tuesday, March 25, 2008 4:20 PM

To: Loyal and Karen
Subject: Re: hi
Hi Karen:

Feeling better every day, slowly getting my energy back.

Here's the good news and the bad news about the doc visit this morning:

Good news: Nothing in the lymph nodes, and the lump was only 5 millimeters! No complications in the healing.

Bad news: The surgeon needs to go back in and take a little more since there wasn't enough margin, or space between the good tissue and the cancerous tissue, at least on one side. She just wants to be sure it's all out since it is the invasive, fast growing type. Surgery will be a week from Friday. It will be easier this time, with only a local.

Good News Again: God is SO in control of this, and I am at peace. I know I am in His hands! Thanks for the prayers!

I am having fun watching the guys put in the sports court down in the back yard. Kids are champing at the bit to go play down there, but we have to wait for the cement to dry. Weather has been perfect for cement drying!

Love!

Shelley

From: Shelley
Sent: Wednesday, March 26, 2008 10:18 AM
To: Gini
Subject: Re: dinner
Hi Gini:

Thanks for the VERY delicious dinner!! Everyone loved it. You are such a good cook. Mrs. Grass's Soup mix, right? I can never remember, but I really need to add that recipe to our cook a lot menus! Plus those divine potatoes.

Let's see what time we'll need to be at the hospital on Friday to decide about Luke spending the night. My mom's been itching for him too. This week Luke and Kristin are having some special times, so I think we're covered there. She goes home Saturday. Then three weeks of school left, then home for the summer for her.

Bible Study next Thursday would be great!! I am a glutton for prayers! (and your food).

Thanks so much!

Shelley

From: Gini and Daniel
Sent: Wednesday, March 19, 2008 8:02 PM
To: Bible Study
Subject: Prayer Time
Hi Bible Study Friends,

You all must have heard by now that our Shelley needs to have more surgery...just a little bit more to remove. Not horrible news, but certainly not everything we'd hoped and prayed for. Thank you Jesus she is doing well in recovery (saw her yesterday and she was up and about, looking way too good for being just out of surgery...). But, the cancer is an icky one...and can recur much too often. So, as Shelley says, we are not about stats, but we are a people of God and His works.

The McNeil household would like to host a dinner and prayer time Thursday evening April 3rd at 6:30 for our Bible Study friends. We of course will pray heartily for Shelley but if you have other concerns that you would like special prayer for, please bring them.

Missing all of you, praying you are having a good Spring Break and a wonderful Easter season. He is risen!

With love, prayers...

Daniel and gini

One day before my second surgery I received a phone call from a nurse from the hospital. She discussed the surgery, and casually said, "Hmm. So, it says here your cancer is "Her plus". That means you'll need chemo.

"No! That can't be right," I protested. "My tumor was really small, like only 5 mm. The surgeon said radiation would take care of it.

"Well, the usual protocol for these kinds of aggressive cancers is chemotherapy. Talk it over with your doctor."

I hung up the phone and burst into tears. My hair! I couldn't lose my hair! And the throwing up? No way, God. This is not happening.

I then proceeded to spend the next hour online researching. The nurse appeared to be right.

Right about then, a couple of folks from our house church came by with a meal for us. I told them what I had just learned and started to cry. They had come at just the right time, as it turned out. After some soothing and prayer, I felt a ton better. After all, I was in God's hand.

From: Shelley
Sent: Wednesday, March 26, 2008 4:46 PM
To: Cami, Gini, Tanya, Vicki, Marlene
Subject: update number I lost count
Hi Ladies:

Just got a follow-up call from a Good Sam nurse. She kind of sprung on me that because of the kind of cancer I have, I'll probably need chemo :(I'm hoping she's wrong, but my gut says she's not (as did the hour in internet research I just did. How did people cope without instant gratification of information?) Prayers needed to make sure the doctors use all the info they have to make good decisions. And more peace, please. Thanks so much, good friends.

Shelley

Oh, and if you get this email before House Church tonight, please pray that I don't bawl my eyes out the whole time! It might chase the new people away!

Sent: Wednesday, March 26, 2008 5:21 PM
To: Shelley
From: Cami
Subject: Re: update number I lost count
Hi Shelley:

Praying for you to feel so close to your Father this evening as you have to give up your own emotions so others can feel welcomed into your home. I hear how desperately you want God's will for your life, your family, your friends and even your house church. You are learning to be selfless in a way right now that is deep and painful. He LOVES you soooooo much. I love you too. :)

From: Shelley
Sent: Thursday, March 27, 2008 9:51 AM
To: Cami
Subject: Re: update number I lost count
Hi Cami:

Things went really well last night...I held it together except during prayer time, but I always cry then anyway. I think the Holy Spirit lets me know He's right there through my tears.

I going to have Andy drive me around today for some errands (he needs the practice) so I'll drop by your dishes.

From: Tanya
Sent: Thursday, March 27, 2008 8:13 AM
To: Shelley
Subject: Re: update number I lost count
Shelley,

I'm praying for you.

I am so blessed by your courage and honesty during this hard time.

Little Daniel has remembered to pray for you daily...these little soldiers are so realistic, consistant and true. All of my kids love you dearly...and are responding to your situation as they would an or a grandma. So, please let us know what you need or want...and we will serve you and your family with a happy heart.

We will be home Sunday.

Tanya

From: Shelley
Sent: Thursday, March 27, 2008 9:45 AM
To: Tanya
Subject: Re: update number I lost count

Hi Tanya:

I'd rather be the aunt than the grandma :)

Tell the kids I'm feeling their prayers. Enjoy your time with family and have a great trip home. It's snowing here (not sticking, just pretty).

Thanks, Tanya

Shelley

From: Shelley
Sent: Thursday, March 27, 2008 9:42 PM
To: Marlene
Subject: Re: update number I lost count
Hi Marlene:
I'm still waiting to get an appt. with the oncologist to confirm what kinds of treatment. Here is the kind of cancer: The tumor was estrogen and progesterone positive (good, because tamoxifen can target those cells to prevent future ones from growing. It was high grade, though. I think that means it reproduces fast.

The invasive cancer cells around the tumor (found during surgery) were estrogen and progesterone negative. They were C-erb B 2 positive 3+. This means the cell is producing tons of a protein that's bad (can't remember why). Proliferative rate was high (fast growing). The invasive cancer part is the reason for chemo. I think the tumor cells won't grow outside the breast, but these will. However, the lymph nodes were negative, so one question I have is if the bad cancer could have sneaked by somewhere anyway, without leaving a trace in the lymph nodes, thus the reason for needing chemo. Lots of questions.

My biggest problem with chemo is the chance of long-lasting effects down the road. I wouldn't mind the whole thing if I knew it meant the cancer was cured once and for all if there were no side effects. And it won't come back.

Thanks, Marlene! I so appreciate emails, they make me feel loved. Strangely enough, I don't appreciate phone calls from relatives as much because I'm too worried about trying not to get them worried. It's hard to keep reassuring them everything will be fine (and they say it too) when I know perfectly well that no-one except God knows this! But the fact that God DOES know the outcome gives me all the peace I need. Plus I'm enjoying a real closeness right now with God as I read Bible verses that are just what I need at the moment. He's really listening!!

I should write all this down in a journal or something, might need it later :)

Shelley

From: Marlene
Sent: Friday, March 28, 2008 9:58 AM
To: Shelley
Subject: Re: chase update
Thanks for explaining the cells. I'm like you, I want to know and understand. Your science knowledge will take you much further than it will me, but I want words and mental pictures.

I'm relieved that you don't mind emails. I've purposely not called your house for many reasons, most of which are that you need rest and peace. Patients with immediate family around don't need a lot of contact from the "outside". This is the time to connect with your family (your husband and kids) without interruption from others. The phone ringing and always bringing the outside world in can be tiring when you're healing from surgery. The constant need to follow-up, follow-up, follow-up with the clinical world is exhausting in itself!

God bless mammograms. It has saved so many lives when caught early. I'm as close as an email (while I'm at work) so feel free to keep those emails coming!!

Much love!

Marlene

From: Shelley
Sent: Friday, March 28, 2008 8:01 PM
To: Mike
Subject: chase update
 Hi Mike:
Wanted to update you: the surgery went well, I'm healing nicely. The good news is the lymph nodes weren't involved at all and the original tumor was only 5 mm. The bad news is I will need another surgery to make sure they got all of the cancer out...it was too close on one side.

Also, they found a different kind of invasive-type cancer adjacent to the tumor...so I may need chemo after all :(Still waiting for an appt. with the doc to determine for sure. Second surgery will be next Friday. I'm finding lots of great Bible verses about healing during my prayer time, I know our Great Healer is taking care of me.

Specific prayer requests: wisdom for doctors, they keep getting surprised by my results. Wisdom for good choices to decide treatment. Keep the loved ones from not getting too worried. Prayer for Kristin: she chose to stay home this spring break to be here with us this week (dear girl), but now she will be driving down to Redding by herself on Saturday, taking a car to bring back her stuff from school in 4 weeks. Protection for her!! and for her spirit as she handles what's going on with me and her depression (which seems better!).

Thanks so much for your prayers, they are SO appreciated.

I can't believe it's snowing right now!

Shelley

From: Eric
Sent: Friday, April 04, 2008 5:03 PM
To: House church
Subject: Update regarding Shelley

Thank you for keeping Shelley in your prayers. She pulled through the surgery just fine today and is now resting in bed. The doctor said everything looked fine (I recall hearing that 2 weeks ago) and we will hear more about the pathology results when we meet with her next Thursday. This surgery was to 'widen the margin' between the cancerous cells (that were removed last time) and clean tissue, with the objective being 4-5mm. So the pathology should not really show anything but, hey, I am no doctor.

This time they used local anesthesia and a really effective sedative so her post-op is much more comfortable (no breathing-tube irritation). And, of course, there are pain pills if/when needed.

We meet with the oncologist next week where we will learn more about the subsequent treatment. We would appreciate your prayers for comfort and to be free of short-term and long-term complications from this part of the treatment.

The kids and I are doing well. We have been very blessed by our dear friends whom I can never thank enough.

May God bless you all.
--
Eric

Lumpectomy number 2 went well. I dutifully ate my graham cracker in recovery afterwards and was home in only a few hours.

But there was more bad news.

From: Shelley
Sent: Friday, April 11, 2008 5:03 PM
To: Cami, Gini, Vicki, Tanya, Marlene
Subject: What are the chances?
Hi Ladies:

Spent a long day visiting doctors today. The good news is my eye doctor says my eyes are doing great!

But I really should buy a lottery ticket....here's why:

Rarely do women my age get breast cancer

Rarely is it caught as early as mine (God!)

Rarely does it become invasive so early

Rarer still, the kind I have (fast spreading)

Rarely does the surgeon need to go back in to get more on one side

Rarely does she take a little extra on the other side "just in case" (God!)

Rarely does the surgeon find even more cancer cells past this wide margin taken the first time (like mine did)

Thus rarely do people need yet a third surgery

Rarely do people need chemo for so small a tumor

If I remember my stats class correctly, that is Rarely to the 9th power...pretty slim chance!

But our God is a rare God who has it all under his control, proving it by how rare this thing is!!

Last (I hope!) surgery, probably a mastectomy, will be in a couple of weeks, then chemo will start about 3 weeks after that. Should I get a blonde, red-headed, or blue wig?

Seriously, I'm doing fine with it all. Still lots of peace. And my surgeon's a Christian!

Shelley

PS: My up-the-hill neighbor's heart is really softening to God! I'm going to go study the Bible with her next week. Pray for Brenda!

From: Eric
Sent: Saturday, April 12, 2008 9:00 AM
To: House Church
Subject: Chase update
As you read this, be reminded that this is all in God's gentle hands.

You may recall that last week Shelley had an additional re-excision surgery, intended to 'widen the margin' between the previously-removed cancerous tumor and surrounding healthy cells. The removed tissue was analyzed this week and we found out that there were additional cancerous cells in the ducts. This is bad news

-- it means that Shelley will undergo another surgery, currently scheduled for Friday, April 24th. The question here is whether she will undergo another re-excision or a mastectomy. The doctor said this is unusual and will be submitting the case to the 'Cancer Board' next Thursday for review; we expect to hear their recommendation next Friday.

Today we also met with the oncologists (ok, one was a radiologist) to understand our chemotherapy and radiation options. There are obviously trade-offs that have short and long-term health implications, with lots of statistics regarding risks. Thankfully God knows what we need to be doing here, so we await His guidance. If Shelley takes the mastectomy route she will not need radiation. The chemo will take somewhere near three months and will likely start in mid-May. And yes, she will need to shop for a wig so she has to decide on a 'look'.

We know you are all praying for us and we also know that God is answering our prayers. Like a loving father He is giving us what we need, not what we want. To get a glimpse into the need that this is accomplishing it would be a great comfort. Please pray that we gain that insight and are obedient to His purpose. And, of course, we would like comfort, calm, and a speedy recovery to health if that can be part of His purpose.

God willing, Shelley insists we continue to have our House Church meet here as usual.

Be blessed!
--
Eric

At another appointment with the surgeon, she told me she could try for another lumpectomy. Maybe she'd get it all this time. Or maybe not. By the time she was done, there would be a pretty big hole. She urged me to get a mastectomy.

"You are too young. Breast cancer in younger women tends to be aggressive, and tends to come back."

Huh? What happened to the 98% cure rate?

I asked about reconstruction. Can a plastic surgeon put in an implant in right after the mastectomy? I don't want to go home looking like, well, you know.

She assured me that reconstruction was done that way all the time. The plastic surgeon could be right there and insert a small temporary implant. Once a week, I would have to go and get an injection to "inflate" this fake boob, or "foob" as I called it. When it was at the right size and my skin was stretched enough, I would have one last surgery to replace the "foob" with a real implant, which would only last 10 years before it needed to be replaced again.

"Any other options?" I asked.

"Yes, some people opt for a tissue transplant. Muscle from their abdomen or back is transferred to the breast site. It's a very big surgery. I don't usually recommend it."

Ok. Decision made. Mastectomy with implant scheduled.

From: Shelley
Sent: Monday, April 26, 2008 9:28 AM
To: Karla
Subject: Re: Hi Shelley
Hi Karla:

I was just logging on to email you! I'm looking forward to seeing all the rest of the plants in place!

Saturday looks like a great day for planting. Will Amador and friend be able to do everything in one day? We already filled the planter boxes, Eric got them all filled up last Saturday. The fence panels are in too, but we'll need to build that add-on shed/chicken yard to block the view coming up the hill. We haven't done the air conditioner panel yet either.

I'm heading back for surgery on Friday, mastectomy this time, then I should be done thrice and for all. Chemo will start in a few weeks (just in time for the wedding!). My sister and I will have fun wig shopping this week. I am still resting peacefully in God's hand, no worries. They are just trying to get the stray cancer cells that keeping showing up beyond the surgery borders.

See you Thursday! All the plants are getting leaves!

Shelley

From: Karla
Sent: Monday, April 26, 2008 10:36 AM
To: Shelley
Subject: Re: Hi Shelley
Shelley,

You are a strong woman! Such a good decision to remove all of it....I know that that is a hard and sometimes a decision not made due to vanity or pride. It totally makes sense. Yes, they should be able to get done in one day.

I want to share this with you....it is the words on a little card that was in my mom's belongings. It is a great reminder that it is all for good, no matter what the package looks like. I find it calming.

God is in control.

He's allowed this to happen.

He's not biting His fingernails.

He's promised to use this for good.

I'll look for the good.

Breathe in Jesus...

Breathe out anxiety.

Cheers,

Karla

From: Eric
Sent: Thursday, April 24, 2008 10:08 PM
To: House Church
Subject: Surgery is Friday -- please pray

I would like to let you all know how we are doing (mostly Shelley, but myself included) and ask for more prayer.

We expected to hear from the Tumor Board last week, where the surgeon was going to present Shelley's unusual case to a group of experts. We never did hear the results, and so we have decided on the mastectomy-option, which is the subject of tomorrow's surgery. This also includes the first phase of reconstruction (two more surgeries to come) now that Shelley has met with the plastic surgeon. There are too many details to share here, but we were glad to hear that silicone is back! With a new hair-do (wig) and b**b-job, I won't know who I married!

This option means radiation is not part of the subsequent treatment (yay!). For the chemotherapy we mutually agreed on 'ACT', which has our vote for least likelihood of long-term risks. It seems ridiculous to think we are making this decision with any control of the outcome, so we will pray for God's protection in the years to come. We really like the oncologist who has been very patient and acts much like the primary physician in terms of coordination and answering all of our questions.

Surgery will start tomorrow at 1PM or so. Please pray for safety, comfort and healing for Shelley and for God's guidance to the medical staff tomorrow. She should be spending Friday night at the hospital and comes home Saturday, barring complications. Sharon and Kristin will be home this weekend, which is a blessing. Sharon goes back Monday but Kristin will be home for the summer.

I have been asked a few times how I am doing, or about Shelley. My only two answers are (1) we are actually doing well, and (2) we have no option but to hang in there. Your prayers are being answered in that we have an unusual sense of calm and submission to God's will in this. It does not seem odd to me but it must to those who ask, particularly those who do not share the faith. Note also that Shelley is being surrounded with friends who are lifting her up daily, and I thank you all for the cards, meals, phone calls and visits. Shelley is truly blessed by your acts of kindness, as am I.

I intend to send out an update tomorrow. I hope I am not

spamming anyone's mail box. This morning I believe God gave me some insight into what he is working on (at least, in me) so if you were praying for this at 7:30 this morning, bless you. I hope to share more next time.

May God bless you all.
--
Eric

I'm not going to lie. The recovery from the mastectomy was hard. I was in a lot of pain for a couple of days, and when they tried to wean me off the morphine onto pills, the nausea took over. I was SO grateful that my husband was there practically non-stop. He made sure I got my pain meds before I needed them, helped me to the bathroom, held the bowl so I could throw up, called the nurse for me. An untold number of things, most of which I can't remember, because I was so out of
it.

From: Eric
Sent: Saturday, April 26, 2008 1:43 PM
To: House Church
Subject: How Shelley is doing after surgery
As I wrote on Thursday I *intended* to send this update Friday, but that did not happen.

What did happen is that Shelley had her surgery as planned and everything went well. It took twice as long as they had estimated because she is young and thus very vascular. I have never heard doctors complain about complications due to being young; I confirmed that Shelley does not mind when they say that. Thank God that He protected Shelley through all the details of yesterday.

The reason I am late with this update is that she is in a lot of pain and wanted me to stay at her bedside through the night. I popped home for a few hours to make sure everything was okay (and yes, it was) and handle a couple of details. The girls are here safely, along with Andy. Luke is being cared for by some dear friends. I expect to be at her side again tonight, and we should be coming home on Sunday. Right now she is on a regimen of pain meds, an anti-nausea drug and muscle relaxants -- in no shape to be traveling or even visiting.

There is so much more I would like to write, but it will have to wait. I will say that your prayers are deeply appreciated, and those for safety, strength and calm were answered in a big way. Keep praying for healing and a release from the pain. We will continue to put this is in God's strong and yet gentle hands.

Thank you for your words of encouragement. They bless Shelley and me in many different ways.
--
Eric

From: Eric
Sent: Sunday, April 27, 2008 6:45 PM
To: House Church
Subject: Shelley is home, and other thoughts

Shelley is home and napping in her own bed. It is good to be home. The kids were very glad to greet her and visit for a short time. Her pain is generally under control, which is good since the pain is suppose to start subsiding little by little after today. Just before we came home she said she was comfortable for the first time, which is excellent progress. I know you have been praying for this.

I wanted to point out how 'this' has blessed us.

-- Shelley said her devotion time with God is much more intimate and meaningful now more than ever.

-- Shelley also said she could only minister to our just-saved neighbor having been in a 'valley', much like our neighbor is. Shelley should write more on this.

-- Both of us have seen our youngest daughter make some really unselfish decisions in light of 'this'.

-- We have enjoyed God's sense of calm through the entire matter. It is tough to explain, but we really do not feel the need to worry.

-- We have also been taught to let our guard down and just let our dear friends and family minister to us. That is a real challenge for us.

-- I have been blessed to hear Shelley utter 'I need you'. It brings tears to my eyes to write this.

-- I have been happy to lay aside my other priorities (including job) and just be there for Shelley. This is usually tough for me, but not now.

-- I have heard encouraging words from so many of you. You all are praying for us, and I know that pleases God as well as blesses us.

-- I get to write prose like this. What more can I say except that I would never do such a thing.

How is God working through this? I believe he is powerful enough to use something negative like breast cancer and use it to change many lives, in many ways. Although this is tough, I believe he is correcting and teaching us through this. Of course I have been praying (and asking for prayer) that His purpose is revealed to me, and I think I received a glimpse on Thursday, and confirmation on Friday. He told me that I have not been obedient to the teaching in Ephesians 6:5-8 and Timothy 6:1 (Friday's devotion) regarding sincere obedience to employers. It is no coincidence that Shelley's condition coincides with some really bad chemistry going on at my work. If it weren't for Shelley and the subsequent need for stable, supportive employment, I would have quit. But God has allowed me to enter a situation where I have to rely on Him and be obedient -- I would quit if I could, but that is not a possibility now. Sure, I have been outwardly respectful of my boss, but not in my heart which He can clearly see. God is gently breaking me of this sin and I am convinced He will keep me there until the job is done. I pray that I do not cause Shelley to suffer needlessly because of this. I humbly ask for prayer for me as God works through this.

We have a lot of doctor's visits over the coming weeks for post-op care, reconstruction, and chemo (probably 3+ more weeks before that starts). Thank you all for your continued prayers. I hope my letter illustrates that God is answering them.

Warmest regards,
--
Eric

From: Marlene
Sent: Monday, April 28, 2008 7:46 AM
To: Eric
Subject: Re: Shelley is home, and other thoughts

Eric:

Thank you for such a wonderful and heartfelt message. I drive along Barrows every day on my commute to and from work. I pray often, but while I'm on that road I listen to my music and pray for all of you while I am in your neighborhood. Please know that you guys are on my mind often throughout the day.

I'm sure it will be awhile before Shelley reads this. Please give her a hug for me, or if a hug isn't possible quite yet which is likely the case, a super big squeeze of the hand. You two are so blessed to be together.

I have yet to hear of a person or couple dealing with these types of life challenges who didn't say later on that they actually found the challenge to be a positive event in their lives. It's hard to imagine that, but when they had to go 'into' themselves to find what were the most important parts of their lives, it wasn't the job, or the house, or the yard, or the cars, or the trip coming up. It was the time to rediscover each other and their loved ones on a much deeper level. Brings many couples and families to a better place. I can see that happening with you and your family.

My love to all of you and continued prayers.

Marlene

From: Eric
Sent: Wednesday, April 30, 2008 9:27 AM
To: Marlene
Subject: Re: Shelley is home, and other thoughts

Hi Marlene,

We have dinner provided tonight and Friday. Let me see how it works out, but Shelley and the kids may appreciate pizza on Thursday. Again, let me get back to you about that. We see the doctor this afternoon where she will be re-dressed. Her pain is mostly in her back, and seems to be muscular, I think because she cannot lay on her side any. She is on pain meds and muscle relaxers, and I have been giving her (gentle) back-rubs but it is still uncomfortable for her. Do you have any advice? She tried a warm-pack but that did not do the job either. Of course, prayer for comfort would be helpful regardless.

Her med's are making it really hard to read (concentrate) on the paper. It is the quality of the material, not the drugs. So she is mostly watching TV between naps. Movies are too long for her since she misses most of the plot and has to re-wind/re-watch. Seems tragic but she actually sees the humor in it. Anyway, if anything comes to mind that would lift her spirits given her 'state' it would be appreciated. Wish I could be more specific.

Thank you for your kindness.
--
Eric

From: Marlene
Sent:Wednesday , April 30, 2008 9:58 AM
To: Eric
Subject: Can I get anything for you?

Yes, I remember how reading was simply not interesting to me when I was on pain meds, but after I was off the meds, it was back to normal.

I know for some patients, just having soothing music is very comforting. In fact, that's why many hospitals have harp players go through the wards. Something soft and soothing. But - not all patients like it.

The trip to the doctor will be absolutely exhausting for her. Have her take a dose of pain meds before she leaves - probably 20-30 minutes prior so it can start working before she gets up and into the car. Even though it will feel good to get outside, just being up and around will take a lot of her energy from her. She may sleep better because her tiredness will be from physical exhaustion rather than drugs. Narcotics can play havoc on our brains. They can keep the pain away at the targeted spot, but create pain in other area's because of limited movement, etc.

That being said, it is key for her to make sure she takes her pain meds as prescribed. She will heal faster, heal better and have fewer long term effects by taking her meds as prescribed, rather than trying to "tough it out". Lots of research to support this. So if she's trying to go longer in between her meds than she should she will suffer much more and her overall healing will take longer.

Lot's of fluids. I just spoke to a nurse who broke her back this last January, and she said lot's of fluids to stay hydrated was very important for her recovery.

She also mentioned Quantum Touch. I don't know anything about it, but it sounds like just gentle touch, the heat and energy of your hand soothing the different areas. This isn't a massage - just a laying of hands for periods of time. I've tried this type of thing before, and the warmth of someone's hands is very soothing, even when you aren't in pain. Give it a try.

Hope I've given you some ideas. Let me know about pizza when you know. God Bless You! You are such a good husband. I will continue to keep all of you in my prayers, especially Shelly's comfort and to be pain free very soon.

Marlene

From: Gini
Sent: Thursday, May 1, 2008 3:43 PM
To: Shelley
Subject: Luke Testing
Shelley,
Not to bug you.... Oh my...

I got the postcard from Basic Skills regarding testing for 3rd grade. I have a call in to them for Luke and Hope and will just sign him up. I'll bring him too...not to worry. It's June 10th,

Tuesday.

Praying, praying, thinking a lot about you...missing my friend.

love,

gini

From: Shelley
Sent: Thursday, May 1, 2008 8:32 PM
To: Gini
Subject: Re:Luke Testing

replying here from drug induced haze..please sign him up. Thanks...
just send me a bill.

This email is takig me 10x longet to write... pretty scary. I justasked
kristin what Bible story was on tv, and I think theywere watching a
bug exterminator showw....Everyone's laughing at me.

Field trip from other email sound great...you'll just have to forgive me
ad give ma a few days notice, maybe earlier in the day when I might
be nearer my calendar...assuming I can still holda pencil. Bergtter
quiit, now while, I'm behing.

aWhlwly

(Eric adds: Shelley wants Luke to participate in both the field trip and
the testing. Please sign him up and we will reimburse you.)

From: Gini
Sent: Friday, May 2, 2008 4:45 PM
To: Shelley
Subject: Re: Luke Testing

Oh my...whatever I can do... I don't know if I should smile or cry.

I'll take care of everything and whatever else you need.

praying even harder!

gini

From: Shelley
Sent: , May 6, 2008 11:57 AM
To: Gini, Tanya, Cami, Marlene, Vicki
Subject: feeling good!

Hi ladies:

Finally off pain meds and starting to feel human again. I'm wearing clothes (sweats are clothes, aren't they?) and not PJ's today! Every day is a little better, and sleeping is now so much better at night. Eric has been so amazing through all of this, I feel very loved. He has been getting up in the middle of the night a couple of times to make sure I had meds ready before I started to need them, giving me sponge baths, fluffing pillows. Plus staying with me the whole time in the hospital. Truly he is one of the most amazing blessings God has shown me. Plus Kristin pitching in and helping with Luke, homeschooling him, and taking him on outings, making meals. Another amazing blessing.

Oh! And Andy got the internship for this summer!!! We are all so excited about that. I am overwhelmed with God's blessings!!!

One drain out, one to go. Then a week or so before chemo starts. Let the fun times roll. Plus only weeks until the wedding!! I think

Sharon and Will are on top of things in that category. If not, the only important part is the "I do's!"

Thanks for the prayers, meals, and listening ears!!

Love,

Shelley

From: Shelley
Sent: Thursday , May 8, 2008 1:09 PM
To: House Church
Subject: good news today
Hi everyone, I'm out of PJ's and onto the sofa with actual clothes!! Feeling better every day, no more painkillers (my family was laughing at me, and I have no memory of doing anything funny!!) Life is good and full of blessings. On the way to the doctor's visit today I noticed and enjoyed all the beautiful flowers in bloom right now and the view from St. Vincent's 8th floor lobby is magnificent with Oregon's fascinating clouds and sunbeams streaming through. How can we not be glorifying this Creator every minute for sharing!!

Good news from the surgeon today, we made the right choice because there was definitely more cancer beyond the first two surgeries, but now there is no evidence of anything left. That means no radiation, just chemo, which will probably start at the end of next week or the beginning of the following week. Finally some good news for a change!

Hope to see some of you on Sunday and at House Church next week!!

From: Jan
Sent: Friday , May 9, 2008 10:30 AM
To: Shelley
Subject: Hey Shelley

Shelley,

Just read where you're doing pretty darn well! I'm SOOOOO glad to hear that! Eric's messages when you were facing surgery, in surgery and barely out of surgery were so touching! God is so Good!

As you well know, many of us have prayed for you and your family – the wedding is another matter of prayer of course (and much praise too)!

Keep on gettin' better and better!

Jan

p.s. Guess what? I'm filling in with Joyful Noise for a few weeks – wow, it's more fun that I thought it would be!

From: Shelley
Sent: Friday, May 9, 2008 11:12 AM
To: Jan
Subject: Re: Hey Shelley
Thanks, Jan! I took my first shower today and I'm feeling so nice and clean!!

Thanks also for doing JN for a few weeks, I know Gini is extremely grateful for a break. It can be pretty overwhelming, as we all know.

Thanks for all the prayers, I am feeling very loved, at peace, and held closely in my Father's Right Hand. Plus, how can you beat breakfast in bed lovingly prepared by a nine year old, complete with cold toast and cereal that slides off the tray onto the floor (where Freddy, the black lab, eagerly awaited). Priceless memories!!

Love,

Shelley

Treatment

From: Shelley
Sent: Monday , May 12, 2008 11:11 AM
To: Gini
Subject: points to ponder
Hi Gini:

Feeling lots better, one week reprieve before chemo (next Tues, I believe). Luke and I are on a mad dash to finish up school...I think we caught up to week 35 this week, so we just might finish before Memorial Day. I KNOW my patience for school will not hold up much past that...but things have been going much better, school-wise, so happier times around here. We will still need to continue to review things before testing (did Luke get signed up? Do I need to do something?).

Don't need anything this week, I'm so glad to be driving again!! I have big helper boys who will help with shopping, laundry and such. Kristin reminded me that SHE started doing her own laundry when Luke was born at age 9. Hmm. I read a devotion yesterday by some famous lady who had breast cancer (was it Billy Graham's wife?) which said her four kids (ages 17-9 maybe?) learned how to help around the house more and become more independent, since mom couldn't control every aspect of their lives anymore. And they discovered just how much there was to do. Yet another blessing to the Chase house, I believe. (Why aren't my magic underwear drawers filling up as usual? Why doesn't the magic refrigerator fill up with milk? And on that subject, what is in that refrigerator that smells so bad?) The great mysteries of life...

Shelley

From: Shelley
Sent: Monday , May 12, 2008 2:23 PM
To: Gini
Subject: Re:points to ponder

Between Eric (the chemo place is right by his work) and my sister, I think I'm covered for any needed rides. I may need a place for Luke to hang out, though, depending on Kristin's work schedule or Caleb's availability (it is right near his house too). Only once every three weeks, at any rate. Thanks!

Summer is soon here!!! 95 degrees on Friday!!! And after about 10 years of homeschooling, and every single year saying we will do "some school" all summer, I have finally figured out everyone needs a summer vacation from school. Especially the teacher. Most emphatically and with ten exclamations points, the teacher.

Prayer request for now is about chemo effects...I've heard the gamut from "really not too bad" to "I was stuck in bed immobile for 10 days after each one." to "I had to quit. Too hard". I've decided to stop reading the computer forums about these (the source for this iffy info) because it was making me fearful, and no way is the enemy going to win at that game. GOD IS SUPREME!! Thanks for the added angelic warriors you are praying into service on my team!!

Shelley

From: Shelley
Sent: Tuesday , May 13, 2008 11:45 AM
To: Tanya
Subject Praying here, Tanya
Hopefully this nice gentle rain will wash some of that bad pollen down out of the air.
One of the devotionals I read this morning was about Peter taking his eyes off of Jesus and glancing down on the water. It was only then his lack of faith caused him to sink. This was a good reminder to me (and you too I hope!) to not look down into the water!! That

water is way too big and scary! Keep those eyes on Jesus and he'll take you one step at a time...

Love,

Shelley

From: Tanya
Sent: Wednesday , May 14, 2008 2:23 PM
To: Shelley
Subject: Re: Praying here, Tanya
Shelley,

Thanks for the encouraging words yesterday. I am focusing on keeping my eyes on the Lord and listening to Him through this. :)

How are you feeling?

Talk soon,

Tanya

From: Shelley
Sent: Wednesday , May 14, 2008 3:02PM
To: Tanya
Subject:
Hi Tanya:

Of course you are! Me, I'm still glancing down at the water occasionally and having fear moments (I've decided not to read anyone else's chemo story. There are too many different side effects with too many variables and everyone is different!!). Pray in a few extra angelic warriors on my side of the team, will ya?

Sharon and I will be able to go to BCC on Saturday morning at 11:30 to meet with wedding coordinator. Did you say you could come? Don't add that to the list if it is going to put you over the top!

I am having times of feeling really good with lots of energy followed by bouts of really tired. Hmmm. might they be related? I think time to re-institute afternoon nap time (for me). I cried about having to take a nap every single day when I was 4. Maybe I've grown up a bit.

Shelley

As it turns out, the actual process of getting the chemo chemicals into your body isn't too bad. I had a port put in during the mastectomy, which is a small device under my skin that a nurse can connect into with a needle to insert an IV tube. That process stings a little, but it is very quick. After that, the nurses can connect all manner of chemicals, one at a time, into your IV tube painlessly and easily. This is a much nicer route than having nurses poke and search for veins every time you go in for chemo, especially when your veins get kind of beaten up by the nasty drugs. When your chemo session is over, the nurse removes the IV tube and you never know it was there.

Once I was hooked up to the chemo, I immediately got a metallic, chemically taste in my mouth. It helped to sip some tea. Since the chemo process takes hours and hours, I was able to eat a little lunch, read, use my laptop, chat with the nurses. Some of the other ladies around me took naps. Afterwards, I had no trouble driving myself home.

From: Shelley
Sent: Wednesday , May 21, 2008 12:11 AM
To: House Church

Subject : Chase update

Hi all:

Just wanted to let everyone know that the first chemo went just fine, although it took a lot longer than we expected. Got there at 10:30 and didn't get home until close to 4:00. Hopefully the next ones (only 5 left!) won't take quite as long. They have wireless internet! so Eric was able to do some work, and I am enjoying a Randy Alcorn fiction (the one on China) which is really good. Next time I could bring my computer and watch a movie.

Feeling good today too, no problems. Because of the steroids they gave me, I couldn't sleep last night from about 2:30 - 6:30, but I hope everyone feels well prayed for today, so it was time well spent. Maybe I can catch a nap later, after a 3:00 doc appt.

Thanks so much for all your prayers. I don't expect it will all be this easy in the coming weeks, but God has laid out the path and I will be walking step-by-step.

A praise and answered prayer from my neighbor Brenda, whom we prayed for at house church. She ended up being in the hospital 8 days, but on one of the days, a nurse came by after she was off duty and brought a Bible. She read to Brenda and they had a little Bible study. The nurse said she felt like it was something she needed to do. So our missed day of Bible Study with Brenda was replaced for us!! I think that is just a totally awesome thing for God to do. She wants to come to church with us in week or two, but her husband Bob wants to go back to the Unitarian church they visited. You prayer warriors know what to do about this one.

blessings,

Shelley

The night after chemo, I always started to feel achy and feverish. My appetite would go away, but I really wasn't feeling sick to my stomach. I didn't even need the anti-nausea medicine.

My intestines, on the other hand, took a big hit every time. The diarrhea started the next day and lasted about 7 to 10 days almost every time. Nothing really seemed to help much. I just needed to stay at home and be near the bathroom. Since I was tired anyway, no big deal. I just rested as much as I could. By the middle of the second week, I started to feel better, and by the third week, usually felt great. Just in time for the next chemo.

As I re-read the emails around this time, it struck me that life went on. Sure, I was not feeling good for a week or so, but other than that, the months of chemotherapy were filled with everyday life and living. There was no need to put everything on hold.

From: Shelley
Sent: Wednesday , May 27, 2008 5:58PM
To: Vicki
Subject Re: Just checking in
Hi Vicki:

Doing great, still have my old hair. Kinda wish that part was over, not knowing which day is "off with it!" day.

Spending a lot of time in "the little room", Immodium may or may not be helping (I guess it could be worse!). But feeling a bit better every day. Today I was able to go outside and plant a few pots. It looks like about a week after each treatment will be "rest period", then I'll have a couple of weeks to play between. If the first time is any kind of predictor, anyway. But so far, very do-able!

I found out today my plastic surgeon has gone through chemo. He was able to work through the whole thing, he said, with maybe only one day off. What a guy. I wouldn't have wanted to be doing surgery last Friday!! "Um could you guys hold this scalpel for a minute while I run to the bathroom?"

Luke is counting the days until Caleb is out of school and can come play. Luke may still be doing school all summer at his current rate. I told him he has to finish the math book and writing book before school is over. He likes to skip or do half a lesson, and it has finally caught up to him!

Hope all is well with you!

Shelley

From: Gini
Sent: Tuesday , June 3, 2008 9:40 Am
To: Shelley
Subject: re: Thurs
Shelley,

I thought that chemo was Tuesday... If it was the same day of the week as last time. Would you like dinner? Since Andy will be home, I won't subject Luke to the ballet ladies but bring him home around 3:30 when I do the carpool pick-up.

I know you must be whacked...the emotional roller coaster is enough to wear out the strongest of us (that would be you) much less the physical trauma you're going through. Did you know that there's this 100 point stress gauge thing?

100 for a move or a re-model,

100 for a wedding,

100 for bad illness,

there's a couple of other items on the list but I wonder what a sister's move and a mom's move would count as? What about a daughter that has need of serious prayer? ...did I mention that you are hosting the reception and doing chemo?

How does it feel to be Job? Eric must be feeling Job like as well.

Praying and praying...with love and looking forward to Thursday.

gini

From: Shelley
Sent: Tuesday , June 3, 2008 8:06 PM
To: Gini
Subject: re: Thurs

Hee, hee: add putting an offer on the property next door this week (and negotiation for it) to the 100 point list! Pending baldness must be about 100 points. What do I win if I get up to 1000 points? Seriously, I am so at peace with everything I'm beginning to think God is spiking my drinks.

My house is better for this embarrassing reason: I still am visiting the bathroom 5-6x/day, no planning ahead. I've been so used to staying home lately because of this, so when you said deck, I just assumed mine! Sorry! Hope you don't mind...

Sharon will probably be home too on chemo day because of a dentist appt (trying to squeeze in one last time on OUR dental plan). She could probably work something out for dinner. You have been so good! Might need it next time!

For this Thursday, Andy gets out of school early and our carpool is bringing him home, so no time constraints. Treats sound good! My appetite has returned full steam ahead. I'll brew the tea, or lemonade (does that need brewing?) or whatever sounds good (might be hot coffee if this weather holds). Maybe even something God has spiked...

See you Thursday!

Shelley

From: Shelley
Sent: Thursday , June 5, 2008 7:27 PM
To: Mike
Subject: check this out
Hi Mike:

Monday's better than Tuesday, Tuesday afternoon is chemo #2 so I'll literally by "tied up" all afternoon. Tuesday morning is OK.

I went to Great Clips this morning and had the hair that hadn't fallen out yet shaved off and the wig put on. The person before me had just complained for 10 minutes about her hair cut, so I made it easy on the hair cutter and told her that I was "pulling a Brittany". I like it better than my old hair (no gray!).

Madly trying to get all the details done for the wedding while I'm feeling good. Going to Seattle this weekend to watch future son-in-law graduate.

Thanks for the offer of help. We're probably set for furniture movers since all the groomsmen will be in town not to mention all 5 of the bridesmaids (who are sleeping here! Good thing the house is bigger!)

From: Shelley
Sent: Thursday , June 5, 2008 7:27 PM
To: Gini, Cami, Tanya
Subject: wedding duties
Hi:

Is there a day next week (Mon, Tues, or Wed) when we can get together to discuss wedding duties? Thanks so much for your help!!

Yesterday was a bed-all-day day (feverish, achy), better today, so it is a sofa-all-day day. I expect to feel better tomorrow. Prayer request: my blood test shows I'm pretty anemic, so I'm going to tank up on iron for awhile and hope I don't need a blood transfusion or the unknown future effects of RBC booster shots. I will know by next Tues or Wednesday if I start to fade away...then I'll have to go in so I can sit up for the wedding. Pray for sun!!

Thanks so much for your prayers! No intestinal side effects to speak of this time!!

 Shelley

From: Shelley
Sent: Thursday , June 23, 2008 10:13 AM
To: Karla
Subject: Wedding weekend

Hi Karla:

The wedding was fantastic, no hitches in the "getting hitched". Sharon was a beautiful bride, and her husband-to-be almost lost it when he first saw her coming down the aisle, but recovered and the ceremony was great! They skipped down the aisle at the end.

The garden was beautiful and we still have some butterflies flying around from the butterfly "release". Most importantly our septic tank didn't clog up or overflow (should have thought of a port-a-potty!). Quite the test for the new system. The reception went very smoothly. It all went by so fast!

Lots of people praying for my energy level, it was pretty low up until Tuesday, but I recovered just fine and had about 4 days of non-stop activity with relatives. Maybe a few relatives left over today even, to visit and eat up left-overs. All great fun! Glad we are done for a couple of years with weddings (although my nieces have already expressed interest in the backyard for their weddings...but they have to find guys first.

Thanks so much for making the yard so beautiful!! Come and take pictures anytime. Or maybe we'll send you some!

  Shelley

From: Shelley
Sent: Sunday , June 29, 2008 8:56 PM
To: Gini
Subject: Re: Just checking in
Hi Gini!

Keeping yourself busy, I see..."Don't put off until tomorrow, just do everything today". Wow. And with company coming!!

It's been a really interesting week, lots of strange side effects. I finally went to the doctor on Friday for my very pimply scalp, she took one look, gasped, and said "OH MY GOD!!" Aren't I special to shock my doctor? She had never seen anything like it. She thinks I might be allergic to the steroids. We're going to try chemo without the steroids this time to see if it would help. That might cause a problem during chemo itself (allergic reaction), but we'll hope for the best. Yay for no steroids!! They make it very hard to sleep after chemo!

Other issues continue, one almost caused me to go to the ER on Friday. Soaked through three sets of pajamas in an hour. I thought chemo was supposed to put me into menopause! I'm doing better now, just really anemic. This will be blood transfusion week, I'm sure. Also chest X ray week (bad cough, low fevers). Oh boy, I'm starting to sound like my dearly departed grandmother, with all this complaining about health issues!! Sorry. Prayers appreciated!

Shelley

From: Shelley
Sent: Thursday , July 10, 2008 10:12 AM
To: Marlene
Subject: Re: Hi!
Hi Marlene:

I am doing fine, had chemo number 3 yesterday. Last week I had a bad cough and low fever, so the doc delayed chemo a week. She also had me do a chest Xray (normal), a CAT scan, an ultrasound (for bleeding) and a uterine biopsy (normal). Also got 2 units of blood. Good grief. Today I get an ultrasound of my thyroid (the CAT scan said something was up, but the doc said these tests usually turn out nothing wrong). I think one test leads to another and it will all be a waste of time in the end. At least Luke is at camp this week so he doesn't have to wait around for me all week. I'm getting all these unusual side effects that the doc has never seen before (aren't I special). This week I am doing so much better, the rash is better, the cough is almost gone, the bleeding is slowing, and I have more energy (thanks to whomever donated blood!!). Things are looking up, and I am now halfway done with chemo. Hurray!

Shelley

From: Shelley
Sent: Sunday , July 23, 2008 11:23 AM
To: Cami
Subject: Re: Check in
Hi Cami:

Sorry I didn't let you know right away..thyroid.biopsy NORMAL!!!! The doctor finally called in the afternoon, right before I went up the hill to do a Bible study with the neighbor. I am so praising on this one!! I was starting to worry a bit, thinking she didn't want to call me and tell me bad news...but it's all good. Thank you, Lord!

Shelley

From: Shelley
Sent:, July 21, 2008 1:41 PM
To: Vicki
Subject: Re: Yikes
I'm at chemo right now. They weren't sure I could have it today since my red blood count was so low...lower than even right before I got the blood transfusion last time! I was very surprised since I don't feel tired at all this time! The doc-on-call (mine is gone now)

wants me to get a shot of red blood cell booster, but I don't like the research on this drug. The FDA says reserve it only for terminal patients, of which I am NOT. It has been shown to increase the risk of breast cancer (ha, ha). I will go for a blood transfusion, maybe next week, instead. Safer.

Shelley

From: Shelley
Sent: Thursday, July 31, 2008 11:30 AM
To: Loyal and Karen
Subject: Re: saying hi
Hanging out on my bed today, just pretty tired, and pretty tired of watching "design my room" shows.

So is that bladder pill orange, and makes pee orange? That did nothing for me when I had my bladder infection a couple of weeks ago. I'm thinking that pill is a waste of a glass of water. And it stains!!!

So glad you can stay home with Karen and entertain her through this rough time. I have Andy home with me today (I didn't want to take him to work, so he called in "My mom's sick".) I've been texting him all morning to be my slave boy. Right now he is taking Freddy for a walk, because that poor dog won't leave my side and he is driving me crazy!! He also did some interesting things to my computer (Andy, not Freddy)...the jury is still out on that.

Love you both lots, and I hope you find some interesting shows on TV other than Dr Phil!!

Shelley

From: Eric
Sent: Sunday, August 24, 2008 3:26 PM
To: House Church
Subject: Update on Shelley, and family
Hi--

Each time I am asked how Shelley is doing I get convicted that I have not sent out an update in a very long time. I am also humbled by how many of you dear friends that lift Shelley (and me) up in prayer, so it is the least I can do to write this short note.

Shelley just had her 5th (of 6) treatment of chemo last Wednesday. The side-effects are general tiredness, trouble staying warm (or cool; weird, huh?) and loss of appetite. Each subsequent treatment results in quicker-acting and more severe fatigue, and the effects are lasting longer -- beyond a week now. God willing, she should have a good Labor Day week and then she goes in for the last round the following week. We ask for prayer that she regains her strength quickly so she can enjoy some mobility before the next round. I see her filling the 'up days' with as much life as can fit, treating them as a gift, so the more the better.

I may have not mentioned it earlier, but the chemo is purely preventative. There is no test for her afterward to see if it was successful since all of the cancer was supposedly removed surgically. So once she is done with chemo, she is done. We will thank God for that day. She does have some reconstructive surgery ahead once she regains her strength. We don't have that scheduled yet and I intend to ask for prayer when that day comes closer.

Andy, Luke and I are managing well with the help of our friends. Andy is now a licensed driver, which means Shelley can send him on errands now (...prayer would be appreciated here). Luke has been spending a lot of time at friends' houses which is a welcome relief to us all, although we miss him sometimes. My personal battle rages on with occasional opportunities to witness, so I feel God's hand in this. David (as he dealt with Saul) is my inspiration.

Once again, thank you very much for your concern, for your prayers, and for the acts of kindness you have given to Shelley and me. We love you all.

Eric

From: Shelley
Sent: Wednesday, August 27, 2008 11:47 AM
To: Cami, Vicki, Gini, Tanya
Subject: Prayers appreciated
Hi all:

Send some extra prayer over this way. I'm still flat out exhausted from last week's chemo, and still dealing with stomach and intestinal issues. Not really eating yet, either (hurrah for losing 10 pounds in one week, umm, I think...). Sharon and Will come tomorrow, we were supposed to go look and pick out wedding pictures/albums. Not going to make it at this rate. Also my niece Breanna moves in with us semi-permanently, probably today. House church is here tonight. Cleaning lady is helping get ready for that, what a blessing.

Don't really have physical needs from anyone, but just crave the prayers. Thanks!

Shelley

From: Shelley
Sent: Friday, September 5, 2008 2:40 PM
To: Cami
Subject: Re: prayer request
Hi Cami:

Andy just walked in the door. He took the car today and came home one period early. Apparently his last class (computers) is too easy for him and the teacher told him to drop it. So he'll be coming home one period early every day! Nothing else good is offered that period. Let's see, how much money are we wasting using only 6/7 of our tuition! Some PCC or maybe Southridge for next year (or earlier), I'm thinking. Just not enough electives at Westside. He is applying for jobs now too.

Anyway, I declared school over for the day for Luke too. We had a good week! No tears! And some fun, hands on stuff!! And we did everything, including some crafts and memorizing a Bible verse!

After my doc appt., which finally happened 30 hours!! after I first called, the doc sent me straight over to the hospital for platelets. Apparently I could have bled to death if I hadn't received some of those fast (and I somehow hurt myself, or whatever). What this means, she said, is reduced or eliminated last chemo, depending on blood tests next Wednesday. Hurray for less chemo!! I had to go back yesterday for 2 units of blood (6 hours!!) which takes me from very very anemic to just anemic. I feel pretty good today! Also, they let me bring Luke in yesterday, so we had a very nice, quiet 2 hours of school while I got blood (my sis brought him late).

Loving the weather and life right now!!

Shelley

From: Shelley
Sent: Thursday, September 11, 2008 9:05 AM
To: Piano group
Subject: Chase update
Hi all:

It's been an interesting past few weeks: the last chemo was really rough, down and out for lots of days, with all the textbook chemo symptoms, some new to me! Last week I went in for a blood test because I was so tired, and had to go right to the hospital for platelets, which were way too low. The following day was also spent getting two units of blood because my red cell count was the lowest it's been. On the plus side, I was able to have Luke with me for part of it, and we did a few hours of uninterrupted school. We accomplished a lot!

Then yesterday was to be my last chemo, but alas, my red cell counts were the same as before the two units of blood last week! Back to the hospital, where I received another unit (6 hours!!). Chemo was postponed due to that and my slowly rising, but not high enough, platelet count. My last chemo should be next week, if blood counts have recovered.

Another issue for prayer: one of the chemo drugs, Herceptin, I am supposed to get every few weeks for a year. This is a new drug, and it directly targets the type of cancer I have, preventing growth of any cancer cells that somehow survive the other chemo drugs. It has few side effects (my hair will grow back!). However, one negative side effect is it affects heart function, reducing the efficiency of some people's hearts. My heart function has decreased 14%, only 2% off from not being able to continue the drug. I'll be re-tested in 6 weeks. It would be great for a healing of this problem, so that I could continue with the Herceptin!

Thanks so much for all your prayers. I am still resting in God's right hand (sometimes resting against my will!), but not my will, but His, be done!

From: Shelley
Sent: Monday, September 22, 2008 12:39M
To: Pam
Subject: Chase update
Hi Pam:

I'm downstairs on the couch today! Improvement over the last three days. Working towards being able to stand up to brush my teeth :) So glad to be done, done, done! (with this phase).

I don't think we need meals at this point. My freezer is bulging right now with dinners from "Dinners Done Right" and other things I made double batches of earlier. After chemo, I don't really eat anything but jello for a week anyway, and Eric and the boys can heat up the freezer meals. Plus my 27 year old niece Breanna is living with us now, and she can help out. Thanks so much for the offer, though!

Thanks for the prayers!! So much appreciated and longed for!!

From: Shelley
Sent: Monday, October 27, 2008 7:36 PM
To: House Church
Subject: Chase update
I stumped the doctor again.

I've been having fevers off and on for the last few weeks, and thinking it was chemo-related, I didn't mention it to my doctor until last week. She noticed that my temporary implant was swollen, and that I might have an infection. Now that she pointed it out to me, I realized that fluid had been building up slowly for several weeks! Now, despite antibiotics, during the last 5 days, I have been growing far faster than Dolly Parton ever dreamed. I was finally able to get in to see the plastic surgeon today, and he was stumped. He asked a colleague, and the colleague said he has seen something like that only twice in 25 years of practice. Once again, I have won the lottery.

Maybe too much info, but all that to say, I'm scheduled for surgery late tomorrow afternoon to find out what is causing the fluid build-up. The temporary implant will be removed if there is an infection, and the surgery to replace it won't be for several months, thus starting the process of reconstruction all over again from the top. So to speak.

It's a quick surgery, and though I spend the night in the hospital, I don't expect a lot of trouble from it. So house church will be held as planned on Wednesday. Eric will be around, but if you don't see me, I'm upstairs in bed watching ER or House or some other medical drama reruns. Although the real thing is much more interesting.

By the way, I was able to find out about my heart function test results, and my heart function is up!! That is pretty unusual, since I didn't go off the drug that causes the problem (this drug is greatly admired for its ability to prevent re-occurrence). So hurray for prayers!! Praise God! Prayers appreciated for fast healing from surgery, no infection, relief from the very annoying cough that continues, and improvement from anemia.

From: Eric
Sent: Wednesday, October 29, 2008 5:38 AM
To: House Church
Subject: Shelley's surgery last night

Greetings-
I only have a few minutes this morning to send this out, so please
excuse its brevity.

Shelley had her surgery last night (at 9pm) and everything went just
fine. It turns out her swelling was due to blood filling the same
cavity that her expander was in, so they removed it (along with the
blood) and will be keeping her in the hospital for a day or two for
observation. She is at St Vincent Hospital, room 816.

Going forward, it will likely be 2 months or so before the
reconstruction process can be re-started. We have found that the
plastic surgeon is an optimist, so we cannot be too sure of the time
frame yet.

Thank you all for your prayers and support.
--
Eric

PS: For those in our house church, I would still like to meet here
tonight.

From: Shelley
Sent: Friday, October 31, 2008 3:03 PM
To: Melissa
Subject: Re: How are you?
Hi Melissa:
You have great timing! I actually just got out of the hospital today.
I went in Tuesday because of extreme swelling and infection of my
expander. The surgeon ended up removing it and a whole pocket
of blood that had formed under and around it. We'll have to start

the reconstruction process all over again in a couple of months after everything settles down. Turns out chemo probably caused the problem since my platelet count was really low at one point. Some blood vessels must have ruptured then.

But I am all done with chemo now, just the one drug (without the bad side effects) every three weeks until next June. I finished about 5 weeks ago, so was just one week short of exchanging the temporary expander for the permanent implant. Sigh. Best laid plans and all that. Now I will just relax and enjoy the holidays!

Hope things are going well for you and yours!

From: Shelley
Sent: Monday, October 31, 2008 3:30 PM
To: House Church
Subject: Chase update
Hi all:

I'm finally home, and I've learned a lot. Hospitals are very noisy, Judge Judy can sometimes be pretty harsh, I know "Just What Not to Wear", I could make a fortune if only I got into the Cash Cab, nurses can make mistakes, hospitals have fire alarms (but you get to stay in bed, your door just gets slammed shut), and doctors make rounds really early in the morning. Unless it is the day you're supposed to go home, then they come after lunch.

The expander is out, along with a whole bunch of blood that was around it, but I got a lot of someone else's blood back, so am now feeling a whole lot better than before. Not in any pain, just tired from playing with the controls on my hospital bed all night. I should be fully recovered by next week. We'll try again with the reconstruction in January.

Thanks for the good wishes and prayers. Much appreciated!! Man may try to point down the road, but my Lord is the driver of the car!! And He is a much better driver than I am!

Shelley

Reconstruction

After the whole failed implant fiasco, I started doing some internet research on other forms of reconstruction. There was something called a "trans-flap" that interested me, mainly because it used your own tissue to form a breast. The surgeon would take a muscle from one side of my abdomen along with some fat and blood vessels, tunnel it all up under the skin and attach it on my chest, forming a breast. A piece of skin from the abdomen would also be attached to cover it all up. The blood vessels would grow and the new tissue and skin would be healthy without putting anything foreign like an implant that would need to be replaced every ten years.

Theoretically, it sounded great! Plus, the plastic surgeon would do a tummy tuck at the same time. It was a pretty major surgery, with a scar from hipbone to hipbone (dwarfing the C section scar I had) and a long recovery.

The success rate for this surgery was reportedly 98%. I decided to play the statistics game once again and go for it. The tummy tuck benefit certainly helped me to decide.

From: Shelley
Sent: Monday, February 9, 2009 11:21 AM
To: Gini
Subject: Surgery tomorrow
Hi Gini:

Hope you had a great anniversary!

My surgery is scheduled for tomorrow, so I won't be able to do co-op this week and probably next too. I'll be in the hospital through the weekend, then probably at home next week. I am SO looking forward to this being done!! Glad to get it over way before spring break, too!

We are set for meals for the next two weeks, so don't worry about us. Eric will probably sent out an update tomorrow night or Wed.

Luke will be at Noah's on Friday night and Caleb's Sat and Sun, so we are pretty much covered with him. He has an assignment sheet of things to do for the next two weeks, and Sharon can help him (she is home during the day). Thank you Lord for the timing and having family home!!

I'll be at St. V's, but I don't expect to want visitors until the pain gets under control, which might not be until the weekend, if at all. I remember walking the halls while I was in labor with Kristin and looking in the rooms and seeing the mothers with their new babies, and thinking, "Beam me to that! I want to skip this part!". So beam me to next week, Scotty!

Hope all is well with your family. Prayers for an uneventful surgery and no complications are requested! Thanks, friend!

Shelley

From: Eric
Sent: Wednesday, February 11, 2008 7:22 AM
To: House Church
Subject: How Shelley's (almost last)surgery went

Hi--
Yesterday Shelley had her reconstructive surgery, and I am pleased to report that it went very smoothly. She is resting as well as can be expected, with only the pain from the surgery which is being managed with the pain medication. So far, I believe God has spared us from any additional trials, which I believe is an answer to prayer.

Her surgery went according to plan -- 6 hours with two surgeons. She will be in the hospital (St. V's) for 4-6 days depending on how quickly she is up and around. Since blood vessels in the skin are involved (which they want to keep open and unconstricted) they are keeping the room at a warm 80 degrees. Tropical, yes, but also tough to sleep in. I know this first-hand.

Thank you all for your prayers, lifting Shelley and our family (and me) up.
--
Eric

From: Shelley
Sent: Monday, February 16, 2009 3:02 PM
To: House Church
Subject: Chase update too long
Hi all! I am happily nestled in my recliner, using the computer Andy fixed up for me, ready to finally give an update on the surgery. God is SO good to help me get back to feeling myself again.

Here are the gory details of the reconstructive surgery. If you would rather not read them (not everyone likes to watch all those medical shows on TV, I realize) skip down to the BLESSINGS part below.

The surgery started on time and took the two surgeons exactly 6 hours (thanks for that time prayer, Tanya!) and went well. I was pretty much helpless in bed, so Eric spent the night. Unfortunately the hospital room temperature had to be kept around 80 degrees so that all the newly attached blood vessels would remain dilated. This was OK by me the first night, but the nurses kept commenting on how hot it was. One said it was like walking into the tropical rainforest exhibit at the zoo. My poor husband! By day 2-3, the temp was really starting to bug me too. I couldn't have any sheets, blankets, socks, or hat and needed a cool cloth. Blessing not to have hair at this point!

On Wednesday, I drank my meals, was unhooked from the IV fluids, and was feeling fine (albeit drugged up), but by the end of 24 hours I started to have intestinal gas pains. They started slow and increased to about every 2-10 minutes for three days. I really felt like I was in labor. This was not fun. On Thursday, I started to loose my appetite and couldn't eat or drink. By Friday morning, I was hooked back up to IV fluids and again IV pain killers for the gas pain (but they don't work for that apparently.) Darn it for remembering that Bible verse about suffering and all its benefits. About this time, I didn't care for any of these benefits, thank you very much.

Friday morning the doc gave the OK to turn down the heat, and that helped me feel a little better. By Saturday morning the gas pains finally subsided and my appetite slowly came back. I was feeling so much better! Here comes the complications part: the newly attached skin is not doing well. The doc will need to do another quick outpatient surgery in about 1 1/2 weeks to correct this. That probably will fix it just fine. Also, I had a pain pump catheter that was inside my abdomen and doing a great job with pain control. On Saturday, as the nurse was slowly pulling it out, suddenly there was a snap. About 2 inches of the catheter was missing inside of me. Apparently this is not a problem, because I have a huge piece of plastic mesh holding me together there anyway. But it's creepy thinking about it. It would look kind of cool on an ultra sound, I'll have to make sure the tech looks there if I need one of those for something. God forbid.

BLESSINGS! Oh, I am overwhelmed with the blessings! Here is only a sampling:
1) My husband. He slept two nights with me in the sauna room, visited three times a day, watched lame 80's movies and remodeling shows without complaining, and yet still managed to

work 6-7 hours every day (new job, you know). Somehow, he found time to do the laundry at home. He walked beside me and behind me (not a pretty sight in a hospital gown!). When God promised me His right hand would hold me up, he gave me my husband to do it very literally. This whole breast cancer thing is not for sissies, but I am very grateful for the renewed relationship with my husband because of it. He is my hero!!

2) My family. Having Sharon and Will (and Breanna!) living with us right now is just fabulous. Sharon held down the fort, heated up the meals, supervised Luke's school work, took him to study at Starbucks (never too early to start doing that, you know), and made sure everyone loaded their dishes into the dishwasher. All while keeping up with her graduate studies. Andy made sure Freddy was fed, using an organized white board check box system (his dad's an engineer). He got himself up, made his own lunch, drove himself to and from school, vacuumed out the car, fixed up my new computer so I can type this, and got himself home by his 10:30 curfew every night. Homework was probably done too, I'm sure. How great is that from a 16 yo boy!! When I arrived home, Freddy was freshly exercised and bathed, and the house spotless. I might have mentioned a few of these details to my nurse on Saturday. She sighed and said, "I feel like such a failure as a mother!" NO! But my family is awesome. I'd rent them out if you needed them, but you can't afford their fee. It's priceless.

3) Friends. Thanks so much for looking out for Luke on Friday, Tanya, and Saturday, Vicki! Sorry about the no visitors thing, but y'all really didn't want to visit me in the sauna with nothing but a thin gown covering up only a part of me. Just not appetite enhancing. Plus I was concentrating on existing. And watching "My House Is Worth What"? I might have missed the end.

3) No hair. This really is a blessing. My hair has just not been growing back at the rate I was led to believe it would. Now I know why. My bald head was cooler in the hospital, and I did not need to wash my hair! A nurse mentioned that one of the other patients was complaining because the hospital didn't have conditioner. I offered to go make her appreciate her hair. Also, since I can only sponge bathe for the next couple of weeks, no hair is a tremendous blessing!

4) A flat stomach. Really. Really. Flat. For the first time in my entire life. I am in awe of my stomach.

5) Suffering. OK, I really hate it, but it is the truth. Suffering through the last week, and at times this whole last year has taught me SO much. I was going to say that breast cancer turned me into a man, but thought that might be in poor taste. I am hoping God will use what I have learned, using me in some way for His kingdom. I know this will all not be for nothing. It is to His good purpose! All Things!!

PRAYERS: Thank you so much for all your prayer support. Knowing your prayers were lifting me up really helped me when I had no words to pray myself. If I might be so bold as to ask for a couple more? It would be great to have the new skin start growing back nicely so I don't need skin grafts. Also, if would be nice to get back to standing up straight as soon as possible, saving those back muscles. I would love to recover from this thing quickly. My heart function needs to stay at least where it is now to keep on the Herceptin until June, when I will be done with that. Also, I would like to just remind the Healer that I don't want to get cancer again, ever, but His will be done. And thank Him for me too!

Probably people with lingering effects of general anesthesia should not be allowed to write updates. But, there you go. Thanks, friends, for your support!!

From: Shelley
Sent: Friday, February 20, 2009 10:39M
To: House Church
Subject: On Courage and Compliancy
When I was in the hospital, they put on these inflatable socks that blow up and down to massage my legs to prevent blood clots. I grew rather tired of these by the third day. They were hot, and I psychologically connected the air in them to the air in my intestines. I talked the nurse into letting me take them off for an hour. She forgot to put them back on. I didn't remind her. They also said walking around would help prevent blood clots. I did as little of that as I could get away with. You want me to actually walk around farther than the bathroom? I was really being kind of naughty about the whole thing.

So fast forward to Tuesday morning, when I woke up with a sore calf. Now I remember the nurses telling me before I came home that if this were to happen, it was blood clot, it was serious, and I needed to go to the ER. I thought they were kidding. I probably pulled a muscle while sleeping. But all day Wednesday, I prayed over and over, "Lord heal me, Lord heal me, Lord heal me". But I still didn't do what the nurses said.

Wednesday morning, my leg was a little worse, and I figured I was due to see the doc soon anyway, so I made an appointment. When I arrived, try as I might to joke him out of being serious, he refused to play along. He checked me over, muttered, "Please, Lord!" (no really, he did!) and stated that I need to go over to the hospital for an ultra sound of my leg. He thought I wasn't in enough pain for a blood clot, but he said, "We take this very seriously. If this travels up to your lung it could be curtains for you." Oh. He said if I had a blood clot he would have to admit me to the hospital again. Oh. This is not good. They'll put those socks back on.

So my sister dropped me off at the east end of the hospital and I found I had to limp all the way to the west end to the ultra sound lab. But that's OK, because I'm supposed to walk around to prevent blood clots, right?

My doc met me in the ultra sound room, which I think unnerved the technician a little. He did find a blood clot, but it looked like it was in a place where we didn't need to worry about it. No treatment needed. Yay! No going back to the hospital.

So on Thursday I had a previously scheduled chemo and my oncologist met me there. She checked on the final results of the ultra sound (did you know everything is computerized now? Instant info!) She was not happy with the final results and informed me that I now needed to give myself blood thinner shots twice a day for two weeks. Say what? And insurance might not pay much, it might cost $1200. I argued back and forth with her on the necessity of this, saying, "but the plastic surgeon said no treatment needed!" But I finally agreed to the treatment. At least I didn't have to go back to the hospital and those socks. While waiting for the prescription, though, I sneakily called the plastic surgeon so he could get me out of this. His nurse said he was in surgery, but she would send him a text.

Hold on. Texting during surgery?!! We can't drive while texting, but you can do surgery and text???!!!

Well, it all turned out in the end. My plastic surgeon called later (hopefully AFTER surgery) and said he concurred with the oncologist. I would have to give myself shots. Inside, I said. No way. Eric will have to do it. The insurance company ended up paying for the shots with only a $35 co-pay, for $2500 worth of medicine. Thanks all you healthy people for chipping in for me! Please keep up on your health insurance premiums!

And I ended up giving myself the shots after all. No big deal. When I was teaching biology, I had to give myself finger pricks as a demonstration on how to do blood typing. Once for each class period! So I stopped being a baby, and just did it.

Here are some of the lessons learned: do what the nurses say. Everything really does apply to even me. I am not the special one that gets out of it. Don't argue with doctors. They probably know what they are doing and can even text while doing it.

Also, I found this verse, just when I needed it:

Lamentations 3:22 Because of the Lord's great love we are not consumed. For His compassions never fail. They are new each morning. Great is Your faithfulness. I say to myself, the Lord is my portion. Therefore I will wait for Him.(NIV)

Prayer requests: I still have the touch up surgery scheduled for next week. Also I would like for this blood clot to go away, and for it not to be "curtains"!

Now it's time to go for a walk.

Shelley

Unfortunately, the transplanted tissue did not take. About two-thirds of it, along with the attached skin, failed to get the proper blood supply, and needed to be removed. The statistics game was no fun anymore.

From: Shelley
Sent: Tuesday, February 24, 2009 9:57AM
To: Cami
Subject: Surgery
Hi Cami:

I'm feeling pretty good, better every day. Just a little discouraged that the first (or should I say 5th) surgery didn't work as well as hoped, and the 6th will have to "make do" with what's available to fix the problem. This means stretching the good skin as much as possible to cover over the bad skin, or else skin grafts. Also, the doc will cut off the dead tissue that didn't have a good blood supply. There might be more of that than we hoped. I am just hoping I have enough breast left after to call it as such.

I know you are praying, thanks so much!

Oh, the surgery is Thursday afternoon. I should be able to go home by 5 or so.

Shelley

From: Eric
Sent: Friday , February 27, 2009 10:48 PM
To: House church
Subject: chase update

Hi--

I brought Shelley home today from the hospital and I wanted to send an update out before my day is over.

Her surgery went well on Thursday -- only 1 1/2 hrs and she awoke with a pain level of "0", alert and without any nausea. It was a blessing to hear her chatting with the nurses as they wheeled her into the room. She was up and walking that evening, and they would have released her if it weren't for the need to set her up with a 'Wound Vac'. What's that, you ask? Read on.

The Dr. had to remove some of the flesh that was attached in the previous surgery since it was not live tissue, and that has left a sizable wound. So they hooked her up to a contraption called a 'Wound Vac' that, get this, applies suction to the wound 24/7 so that the surrounding flesh holds together and heals. I will spare you any more gory details. The 'thorn in her flesh' is now a box the size and weight of a hardback book, tethered to her via a hose with a nice shoulder-strap. The Dr. says she gets to wear it for 1-3 months, depending on how fast she heals. She is not happy with this arrangement, and please pray that she keeps her mind on how great it will be to shed that thing when the blessed day comes.

Upside? I see the nurses really starting to commiserate with her now that she is a 'regular', and I pray that they are drawn to Shelley's source of strength. That goes for her Dr. as well, who told me his is losing sleep over this case. I know this is in God's hands and so I have no interest in blaming him for Shelley's predicament. Pray we get the chance to explain that to him someday. I know we will be more opportunities since she will have skin graft surgery in the future, and likely another surgery after that. Praise God for good health insurance!

Thank you all for your kind notes, your prayers, and your offers for help. We are truly blessed to be surrounded with good friends and family.

--

Eric

I have always hated carrying a purse. Now I have to carry a big 3-4 pound purse around everywhere I go because it is attached to me.

The surgeon needed to remove about a third of the transplanted tissue that had died, which left a pretty big hole. He put in a wound vac, which is exactly as gross as it sounds. This thing is supposed to apply suction to the wound which somehow makes it heal faster. (10 years ago I might have had to stay in the hospital for months while the hole healed, so I am glad I'm in the now.) I'll need to get dressings changed 3 times a week by a home care nurse, make sure the vac is working, fix it if it beeps, call the repair guy to come over if I can't, charge it every night, basically I came home from the hospital with a new baby. This is supposed to take 1-3 MONTHS to heal. At least it sleeps through the night.

After the hole heals enough, I'll need skin grafts to cover it. Then we'll have to see what can be done to repair the reconstruction job enough to call it quits. One step at a time, though.

I would just like to whine a bit about this. If it can go wrong, it will, Murphy's law, seems to apply to my whole breast cancer struggle. I can count 9 things that have gone haywire in the last year, things everyone says only happen rarely. Or they have never seen it happen before at all. But I also have seen God heal every last one of those things, eventually. I'm not sure my story is an encouragement to anyone who might go through this in the future because of everything that went wrong. But on the other hand, I've got no sign of a recurrence. I am trusting God that the cancer is gone. He promised to walk by my side, and He has. So like Job, I will not "curse God and die", as his wife suggested, but instead thank God for healing each of the issues that have come and gone. He is the Creator and I have no right to question Him about his ways.

Lamentations 3:32-33 Though he brings grief, he will show compassion, so great is his unfailing love. For he does not willingly bring affliction or grief to the children of men. NIV
Lamentations 3:55-58 I called on your name, O LORD, from the depths of the pit. You heard my plea: Do not close your ears to my cry for relief. You came near when I called you, and you said, "Do not fear. O Lord, you took up my case; you redeemed my life.NIV"

Prayer requests: No infection and fast healing. Pain relief. That things will go right for a change. Pray for my surgeon, he's troubled by what's happened. Pray for opportunities to share. Pray for my spirits to be uplifted.

From: Shelley
Sent: Sunday, Mar 2, 2009, at 1:52 PM
To: Gini
Subject: Re:Just call me Murphy
Hi Gini:

Thankfully God spared me the details of the future. He is just taking me one day at a time, but every day. Something that seems really hard to do one day is not so bad the next (are you kidding me? Shots twice a day for how long? 1-2 hour long bandage changes three times a week for 1-3 MONTHS!! No way! Blood tests weekly? Blood thinners for 6 MONTHS!!?), but now I've conquered each of those fears and disappointments. Please, sir, may I have some more? Bring it!!! I know it will not be more than I can handle, with

God.

I don't really need anything. Eric's taking good care of me and my chores, and the kids are stepping up. I guess the hardest part is just waiting for life to return to normal, but it looks like we are months away from that. In the meantime, I have had to drop all pride...dragging a bloody hose around in church, not being able to wear a bra and being extremely unbalanced, not having my hair re-grow, just feeling generally unattractive. Also not being able to get out and garden. Can't really do any projects, I have to be careful not to hurt myself (blood thinners), and I tend to hurt myself a lot doing projects. Plus I can't lift anything. So I'm going to read more. Watch more TV. I can probably ride the exercise bike once my last drain is out and my abdomen is healed more.

But wait, God has given me a couple of projects. My neighbor still wants to meet for Bible Study. Another neighbor just found out her husband wants a divorce, so she will need some prayer (my heart aches for her!). I'm sure he'll give me more to do. And I will have lots more time to spend with Him if I can't run around and do things I normally do to fill the time.

Thanks for letting me vent. I vent better in writing.

Planning on Hope for co-op this week. We'll be cutting out the little books and filling them in. There aren't any fun projects to do with this chapter. Next year's science will be a lot more fun. Next year will be more fun.

Shelley

Hi Connie:

The doc had to remove about 2/3 of what he moved into place.
From my perspective (and the mirror's) I am better off than I was,
but pretty much don't have anything to call a "girl". So after I am
healed up and the skin grafts have taken and are strong, then I'll
have to decide either to call it quits and use an
artificial "supplement" or try again, perhaps with a small implant.
I'm leaning toward the former right now.

 I have some hair now! I've eschewed a hat/scarf today for the first
time.

Shelley's Facebook Status update
3 March 2009 at 09:09

Let's see: My hair has grown 3/4 inch in 6 months, which means a
growth rate of 1/8 in. per month. That means it will be roughly 3
inches long in November of 2010. I figure that's when I'll need my
first hair cut. I had my last hair cut in April of 2008 (not counting the
Brittany Spears head shave in June). So I've missed 5 hair cuts
already. I'll miss 11 more haircuts between now and November
2010. At $30 each, that adds up to (gets out phone calculator) a
whopping $480 savings!! Add in shampoo, conditioner, hair mousse
(I used A LOT of this), home hair dye (ahem, only a little of this), I
might save a total of $550!! I would schedule a trip to the mall (or
at least to my computer) to shop, but that amount of money is

exactly Kristin's college expenses (not counting tuition) for one month. So never mind.

Shelley's Facebook Status update
March 7, 2009
John 14:27
Peace I leave with you; my peace I give you. I do not give to you as the world gives. Do not let your hearts be troubled and do not be afraid.

Shelley's Facebook Status update
March 8, 2009

Remember yesterday's Bible verse? About not being afraid? I didn't realize it was not just for the people on my prayer list!!

Eric's job was eliminated yesterday. The small company where he has worked for only 3 months decided it really didn't need his position after all. Because of the size of the company (10 people), there will be no severance pay and COBRA does not apply. This means as of April 1st we will not have health insurance.

God will provide. Eric and I have no doubt about that. So prayer request simply put: Eric needs a new job, and we somehow need to get health insurance. Or whatever God's will is.

I am so thankful for yesterday's Bible verse coming to me at just the right time, and also this one, which just "happened" to be in the chapter I'm on: Isaiah 12:2 Surely God is my salvation; I will trust and not be afraid. The LORD, the LORD, is my strength and my song; he has become my salvation."

Thanks for praying friends!!

From: Eric
Sent: Monday, March 9, 2008 1:26 PM
To: House Church
Subject: Brief Update - answer to prayer

 Hi-
For those who weren't on Shelley's list, I lost my job last Friday. Too
many details to share; clearly this is in God's hands and Shelley and I
are doing our best to trust all of this to Him. Part of 'this', as she
wrote on Saturday, is that our insurance situation looked bleak.
The good news is that God has answered your (and our) prayers and
it looks like we can continue through this October, and only paying
35% of the premium (courtesy the government stimulus plan).
Praise God!

My search has just begun. Thank you for lifting me up.
--
Eric

Shelley's Facebook status Thursday April 30 2009 update

Heat and Drought

In the course of my reading today, I came across Jeremiah 17:7-9

 "But blessed is the man who trusts in the LORD,
whose confidence is in him.

 He will be like a tree planted by the water
that sends out its roots by the stream.
It does not fear when heat comes;
its leaves are always green.
It has no worries in a year of drought

and never fails to bear fruit."

What struck me is this: We are not promised no heat and no drought!! Just that He will get us through the heat and the drought just fine. Since this has been a year of heat (cancer) and drought (no job) for our family, this brings me great comfort. Thank you LORD!

Shelley

From: Shelley
Sent: Mon, Mar 16, 2009 at 3:53 PM
To: Gini
Subject: Re: Hi friend
Hi Gini:

If you want to skip co-op this week, that is OK with me, but we need to keep up with the reading. Next week is spring break, so we are "breaking". Then co-op here the following week? We can do all the experiments we've missed in one mass effort. It does depend on skin graft surgery coming up, but I won't know when that is until next Monday at the earliest. Bother all this medical junk. I can't wait until its all over.

I'm feeling fine, just tired. Had to stay up most of last night with an alarm that kept going off with my wound vac. I think I eventually starting fixing it in my sleep. The skills I'm learning...

Hair is exactly the same length with no growth, in my opinion, but I don't really care anymore. See, I'm learning! Only important things matter!

Hope you had a nice time with all that family!! Now there's something that really does matter!!

Shelley

...for no other reason than as a reminder to pray. Eric is networking, "doing lunch", sending out resumes, etc., but no response from anything or anyone. I know God has a plan for his job situation, but he's not sharing it for now. We can wait on the Lord though. I know all the Bible verses about God's provision and all that. He won't let us down.

My healing continues, though it has slowed down quite a bit. I have named my wound vac "Edward" (after the vampire in Twilight), and he can be quite noisy at times, but we've gotten used to each other. Edward is making me anemic, but my energy level is pretty good. The nurses come every other day to change the dressing, which takes about an hour and a half. My blood thinner level is checked weekly and it finally has stabilized. I have baby hair now, not real hair. It is a silver/brown color with lots of gray. I'm still thin on top, but all the better to feel the spring sun on my head. God says:

Even to your old age and gray hairs
   I am he, I am he who will sustain you.
   I have made you and I will carry you;
   I will sustain you and I will rescue you. Is 46:4

So I'm not going to complain anymore about the gray hairs.

One prayer request is my wildly fluctuating blood pressure. I believe I have developed "white coat syndrome". Lately when a nurse comes to take my blood pressure, or I get it checked at the doctor's office, it has skyrocketed. So as a scientific research project, I started taking my blood pressure at home at various times of the day. The home blood pressure monitor tells me my pressure is fine most of the time. Not much stress in my life right now (I'm kidding here) so go figure. And salt really does make your blood pressure go up! Chips and Salsa at Chevy's proved that little fact.

Can I just say, life has become so precious? I am enjoying every single day. I'm not taking things for granted as much, and I truly appreciate the blessings of the day. I also have started to pay attention to strangers more. I've been looking for opportunities to help out someone that needs help. Before I was so wrapped up in my own business and life, that I really didn't notice other people around me as I went about my day. Thanks Lord for opening up my eyes. I know You are caring about all those people. There is a song on the radio called, "Give Me Your Eyes" by Brandon Heath that says it for me.

Thanks so much for your continued prayers for our family!

Shelley

It has been eight months since my last chemo, so by now I should have the thick crop of curly hair that everyone gets after chemo. Whatever they had before chemo, it seems most people have hair that comes in curly, often a different texture or color than before. Eventually, most people's hair then returns to their former glory, or lack thereof.

Most people.

My hair before chemo was super thick and curly. Every person who had ever cut my hair before last year had remarked how lucky I was to have so much hair. It was the one part of me that I could say I honestly loved.

Now, eight months later, my hair was about 1/2 inch long, straight, and baby fine. I had very typical male pattern baldness on the top and back where very little hair re-grew.

So back to the internet I went, and it didn't take long to find out that one of the chemo drugs I had been on is known for causing permanent hair damage in about three percent of people.

Yes, folks, three percent. One again I had won the lottery.

I once heard someone say they would rather die than go through chemotherapy. They didn't want to temporarily lose their hair.

Are you kidding me? I would SO much rather live. Even if my hair NEVER regrew.

Now, five years later, my baby hair is longer, curly and thin. I'm still pretty bald on top. But I'm alive. And I have a pretty awesome assortment of
hats.

From: Shelley
Sent: Tue, May 26, 2009 at 9:25 PM
To: House Church
Subject: Chase Prayer request
Seventh surgery tomorrow

In the Bible, seven is a very important number, symbolizing fullness or completeness. I came across these interesting facts on the internet (where, of course, everything you read is true):

In the Bible, Seven occurs 287 times, or 7 x 41.

"Seventh," the fractional part, occurs 98 times, or 7 x 14.

"Seven-fold," occurs 7 times.

The above three numbers together are of course a multiple of seven, but a very remarkable one, 287 + 98 + 7 = 392, and 392 is 72 + 73, or 8 times the square of seven (72 x 8).

Amazing God Mathematics.

More importantly for me though is this: in Hebrew, seven (shevah) is from the root (savah), to be full or satisfied, have enough of.

This is exactly how I feel about my seventh surgery tomorrow. I have had enough of them!

So I would really like some prayer, that none of the things that have gone wrong in the past surgeries will go wrong this time. To refresh your memories, here is a list of some (but not all) of the things that I would NOT like to have happen tomorrow, as in the past:

5 hour delay for the start of surgery, uncontrollable pain after surgery, unexplained bleeding, fever, vomiting, low blood pressure, high blood pressure, infection, blood clot, tubes breaking off inside of me, IV getting clogged, getting a wound vac, wrong timing of a flu shot, and having to stay overnight unexpectedly without a toothbrush. Or a hair brush. But, then again I don't really NEED a hairbrush yet.

So, anyway, please pray that all goes as planned, I come home tomorrow, and this is, indeed, the fully satisfied SEVEN.

Thanks!

Shelley's Facebook post Friday May 1, 2009:

Ode to Edward: An Epitaph

Edward, oh Edward, my wound vac vampire friend
You have been at my side so faithfully lo these last 66 days (but who's counting?)
I will miss your urgent beeping and gurgling,
your requests for new canisters, for unblocked tubing, your hunger for my blood
How will I endure those quiet moments during prayer at church, not having to press "audio pause" at the first signs of trouble?
How will I fill my 6 new hours of free time per week, with no nurses to chat with during the long dressing changes?
How will I go on with my life's journey without your sweet tubing catching on every knob, every latch, every chair and yanking me back into reality?
 Edward, Oh Edward, I know you will pass on to a new love, making their wounds heal faster, forgetting me in your never satiated hunger.
I bid you farewell, forever, and I rest in my faith (and unbridled joy!) that I will not see thee again in this life or the next.
Good bye.

From: Eric
Sent: **Thursday, May 28, 2009 at 9:22 PM**
To: House Church
Subject: Surgery #7 is behind us
Hi--
I wanted to send a brief note since I know many of you are holding Shelley in your prayers.

Her surgery went very well today, lacking any complications that we are aware of. According to the doctor she should not need any more surgeries 'for a long time'. I really wanted to pin down what he meant exactly, but that seemed senseless. I believe he did the best of his abilities (and maybe even better with some Divine guidance) and once again Shelley's health is in God's hands. She is resting in her own bed and enjoying the latest in pain medication. Any nausea seems under control as well.

Small amount of detail: She had the IV 'port' removed that they installed over a year ago, she had the former 'wound vac' site completely sown up, and (how best to put this?) she had some work done to balance things out a little. A bit much for one hospital visit, taking close to 3 hours, but again this should be the last surgery for 'a long time'.

Thank you all for your prayers, for Shelley and for me. I so look forward to sharing how God is answering your prayers that I find employment. No progress is apparent to these human eyes, but I rest assured that He is faithful and will provide exactly what I need.

Deeply blessed,
--
Eric

From: Shelley
Sent: Fri, May 29, 2009 at 6:58 PM
To: House Church
Subject: Harp and Lyre Lessons to Start

I "randomly" turned to this verse on Wednesday before my surgery:

Psalm 71:20-24

Though you have made me see troubles, many and bitter,
   you will restore my life again;
   from the depths of the earth
   you will again bring me up.

You will increase my honor
   and comfort me once again.

I will praise you with the harp
   for your faithfulness, O my God;
   I will sing praise to you with the lyre,
   O Holy One of Israel.

My lips will shout for joy
   when I sing praise to you—
   I, whom you have redeemed.

My tongue will tell of your righteous acts
   all day long,

It seems that everything is healing as it should, no gaping holes, no infections, no problems this time! I am so grateful for everyone's prayers and for God's healing hand in this year of "troubles". After two failed reconstructions, it seems that my scars are to going to remain, but I am glad of these reminder scars, so that I will not forget how God has walked by my side, holding tightly to my right hand, the past 15 months. My renewed relationship with Him, my family, my friends will not soon be forgotten. And for the joy, despite the "troubles", thank You!

Feeling very blessed,

Shelley

A note on faith and re-occurrence:

A year or so after I completed treatments, I started to get a nagging fear in the back of my mind. What if the cancer comes back?

As it turns out, there aren't any follow-up scans to see if the cancer has returned. For a year or so, the oncologist would do blood tests looking for unusual signs of liver damage and the like. I still get mammograms (on one side). Other than that, the only way to know if my cancer has returned is unusual pain somewhere.

So, whenever I had pain, be it a headache, strained muscle, back pain, whatever, guess where my mind went first?

This fear wasn't constant, it didn't freak me out, but neverless, there it was. Ruining a perfectly good day.

After much prayer about this, and asking others to pray, and reading about the sovereignty of God in His word, I finally realized something. God is in control of this. I can do nothing. So why worry?

Fear gone.

And if cancer does return someday, as it does for many people with breast cancer, then we'll deal with it then. God's right hand held me up the first time. He can do it again. Here's what the Bible says:

2 Corinthians 5:1-10:

For we know that if the earthly tent we live in is destroyed, we have a building from God, an eternal house in heaven, not built by human hands. Meanwhile we groan, longing to be clothed instead with our heavenly dwelling, because when we are clothed, we will not be found naked. For while we are in this tent, we groan and are burdened, because we do not wish to be unclothed but to be clothed instead with our heavenly dwelling, so that what is mortal may be swallowed up by life. Now the one who has fashioned us for this very purpose is God, who has given us the Spirit as a deposit, guaranteeing what is to come.

Therefore we are always confident and know that as long as we are at home in the body we are away from the Lord. For we live by faith, not by sight. We are confident, I say, and would prefer to be away from the body and at home with the Lord. So we make it our goal to please him, whether we are at home in the body or away from it. For we must all appear before the judgment seat of Christ, so that each of us may receive what is due us for the things done while in the body, whether good or bad.
NIV

Someone posted these questions on a homeschool forum online that I read a couple of years ago. I felt I needed to answer them.

Question: I've been struck with some severe health problems that will not be resolved for probably several months, perhaps even much longer. If you (or someone you are close to) have ever experienced that, could you please share any wisdom/advice/etc? Thank you.

Answer:

I was not myself for about two years, dealing with surgeries, chemo, more surgeries, complications etc. I learned SO much during those two years! It was a gift...one I never, never would have thought to ask for, but am so glad I received. Here are some things I learned:
1.My outer beauty is not important. Really. I have no vanity left. Inner beauty, defined as how you treat others, how you respond to stress, how you hold up when there is nothing left of you to hold up, that is your beauty.
2. God is my fortress and my strength. When I was most worried

about the future, He gave me peace. He allowed me to come very close to Him when I needed Him. He let me know that if I were to die, it would be OK...because He loves my family, my precious children, much more than I do.

3. My husband is more than capable of running a household. He stepped up and stepped in. Our relationship is closer now than ever before. He is my hero.

4. Take one day at a time. This will not last forever. So don't worry about what is not getting done. Just get through this day. Let all expectations go about what is necessary to do, and just be still.

5. Your kids, even the small ones, can learn to do a whole lot more than you think. And it's very good for them to do so.

6. Life is very precious. Each and every day. You are not wasting it by resting and cuddling kids. And since complaining doesn't make anyone happier, including yourself, don't.

7. It is hard to let other people do things for you. It is humbling, and takes away your control of a situation. But that is a good thing. For you and for the person you allow to help. Don't deny them that pleasure!

Oh, so many more things I learned. But here's the big take-home: Suffering improves you, makes you a better person. It brings you closer to your creator and to your loved ones. Consider it joy!

Shelley
Breast cancer survivor, two 1/2 years and counting

Here's another question:

I know this was discussed a while back. Today I got a reminder in the mail for my "yearly" mammogram. I am going to be 43 in

November. I had my first baseline last September. All negative.

I know there are new guidelines now. I am afraid of all that radiation though as well. But then I am afraid if I don't get one, they may miss something. Also, I don't know if I can handle the stress of a false positive.

I have no history of BC in my family other then my grandmother's sister.

So, do I go by the new guidelines and get one at 50? Or, do I get one every year?

Do the benefits outweigh the risks?

Any opinions on this?

Answer:

I had breast cancer two years ago, at 45. There is NO breast cancer in any family members going back as far as I know, and I have no other risk factors, breastfed all 4 of my kids for years, etc. I went a year and a half without a mammogram (I put it off), and then they ended up finding an aggressive tumor, small, but fast growing. If I had not had the mammo when I did, I would be dead now. See, in younger women (below age 50), the kind of breast cancer found is usually the aggressive, harder to kill kind. The radiation dose from a mammogram is about 0.7 mSv, which is about the same as the average person receives from background radiation in three months. Catching breast cancer early means a high survival rate. And there are NO symptoms to most breast cancer. I could not even feel my tumor (5 mm).

As for not being able to handle a false positive, yes, you will. You will handle it for the sake of being alive for your kids and your grandkids. The biopsies, MRI's, chemotherapy, NONE of it is too much to handle. You will handle it just fine. For them.

Please ladies, if you are over 40, get a mammogram every year.

About the Author:

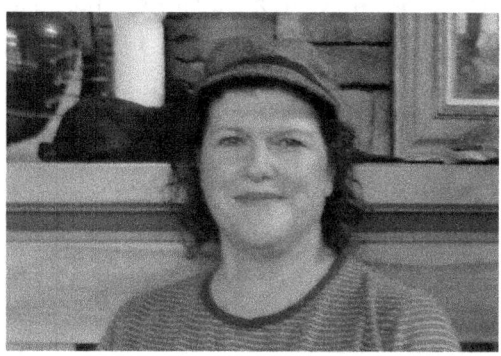

Shelley Chase became a Christian at age 11, praying a simple prayer while kneeling over a hay bale on the farm she grew up on. She lives in the Pacific Northwest with her husband, four children, and one grandson.

Other books by this author available on Amazon:

Signaveria: *Two years ago many millions of people around the world disappeared in what the government called the most horrific terrorist attack in the history of mankind. Sixteen year old Karis's grandfather was one of those who disappeared, but now she and her family know the truth, and terrorists were not to blame. Karis and her family and friends struggle to survive in a world where they are suddenly forced to choose a side, and making the wrong choice can have eternal consequences.*

Michelle's Story: Once Woman's Escape from a Lifetime of Abuse: After a childhood of horrific physical and sexual abuse by her mother and step-father, Michelle escapes this upbringing by getting married young. Her first husband, and then her second husband end up abusing her also. Later on, both her surviving children were abused, one by her ex husband, another by a trusted boyfriend.

Michelle finally manages to free herself from this cycle of abuse. This is her true story of her escape. It is Michelle's hope that her story will encourage others who are trapped in abuse to seek freedom.

www.ingramcontent.com/pod-product-compliance
Lightning Source LLC
Chambersburg PA
CBHW070928290526
45795CB00001B/472